HUMAN REPRODUCTIVE BEHAVIORS

STEVEN HEDLESKY, MD

CONTENTS

INTRODUCTION

We sleep in separate rooms, we have dinner apart, and we take separate vacations. We're doing everything we can to keep our marriage together.

— RODNEY DANGERFIELD

Professional comedians tell us nothing can be funny unless it contains a valid premise. Will Rogers said, "I have always noticed that people will never laugh at anything that is not based on truth."

We can all identify with Rodney Dangerfield's remark because we know human beings do not easily live together in long-term relationships. After a few years, most couples settle into a state of chronic conflict. I have done that twice, through two marriages, each lasting more than a decade before ending in divorce despite our best efforts to stay together. I am now convinced that humans are not meant to be lifelong couples. We try desperately to pretend we are monogamous, but it is just too hard to do.

This is a complete rewrite of human sexuality based on a few basic principles. The first is that, despite our modern cultures, we are still primitive creatures at heart. The reproductive instincts that drive our emotions evolved in the stone ages and have not had time to change. The second is that, during the stone ages, humans did not know the relationship between sex and babies. Human sexuality has been developing along its current trajectory for a million years, but the sex-pregnancy connection was not discovered until people domesticated animals about 7000 years ago. Finally, humans are unique among animals for many reasons, including that they use sex primarily for non-reproductive purposes. Only a tiny fraction of copulations result in pregnancy in humans.

Discard all your previous notions of human sexual relationships. Starting with a few basic biological principles, we will explore why we behave the way we do toward one another. We are primitive creatures living in a modern world of our own making, and our basic mating instincts are in constant conflict with the needs of modern society.

When I say primitive, I am referring to our stone-age ancestors, those humans who lived before recorded time. Conversely, if you prefer, I refer to the time before we were cast out of the Garden of Eden, before we understood the relationship between sex and babies. The term also denotes modern indigenous peoples who have not yet fully emerged from stone-age cultures and retain their traditional sexual and reproductive behaviors. Throughout the book, I purposely avoid the controversy between evolution and creation. I use the two concepts interchangeably, sometimes referring to how humans evolved and at other times to how they are designed.

I must also define monogamy, because the meaning has been modified during my lifetime. Today, sociologists talk about social monogamy, sexual monogamy, genetic monogamy, financial monogamy, serial monogamy, activity monogamy, and perhaps more. This is all very confusing. I am talking about two persons staying together, excluding all others, for a lifetime, "until death do us part." I am referring to the Christian marriage vow variety of monogamy.

I am an emergency room physician. The ER is a unique social

environment. No one is surprised by anything, and every aspect of human behavior is fair game for casual conversation. As an ER doc working the night shift in a small southern city, I have spent countless hours discussing peoples' reproductive behaviors and private lives. I will share some of them with you. These are average people, not urban sexual adventurers. They are surprising in ways that reveal the true nature of human sexuality.

This subject matter naturally divides into three sections. Chapters one through eight discuss the emotional bonds between two people when they form a pair. I focus on heterosexual couples for simplicity of language, but everything in these chapters applies equally well to same-sex relationships. I argue against the notion of humans as monogamous creatures and instead adopt the concept of pair-bonding. In humans, this is a temporary bond lasting four to seven years. It begins with the process known as "falling in love" and ends with the inevitable process of falling out of love. I discuss the emotional components and social mechanics of romantic, post-romantic, and non-romantic relationships.

Chapters nine through twelve deal with the social aspects of reproductive pairing. Marriage is reviewed from the earliest primate pair bonds through human pre-history and continuing through the Mesolithic, Neolithic, and modern ages. The politics of inheritance are a crucial part of this history, and a large part of this section is dedicated to the conflict between men and women regarding the control of paternity. In particular, I include a chapter dedicated to the female orgasm and its role in paternity, society, politics, religion, and war.

Chapters thirteen and fourteen cover sexual diversity with a mathematical analysis. Homosexuality and bisexuality can be explained in terms of population statistics. Inherited behaviors are spread out over standard distribution curves, and some people fall, by chance, into overlapping areas outside of the two sexes or between genders. This is the source of the diversity and versatility that defines the spectrum of human sexuality. Similar sexual diversity exists elsewhere in the animal kingdom: there is no logical basis for labeling homosexuality as unnatural. As with any other characteristic of a population, sexual diversity and homosexuality exist because they provide reproductive advantages.

I urge everyone to read the two appendices. The first contains a series of "why" questions about human sexual behaviors, with answers in a novel analytical format that I find very useful for resolving difficult questions. The second is a collection of jokes that reveal the true nature of human sexuality.

I hope this book will help readers understand their own behaviors and emotions better. We can all learn to deal more effectively with the conflicts we feel when our primitive instincts collide with the needs of contemporary society. Those conflicts cause feelings of shame, guilt, and resentment that lead to unnecessary abandonment of relationships. A better understanding of sexual behavior will help couples reinforce their bonds as they transition into stable long-term relationships.

I also hope this book will convince readers that homosexual and bisexual pairings are no different from heterosexual pairings. All forms of romantic love play legitimate roles in continuing the human species. Sexual diversity has value and should be appreciated.

To resolve the conflicts between our emotions and the needs of our modern cultures, we must first understand the origins of those emotions. To become what we want to be, we must first know who we are.

CHAPTER ONE

BASIC HUMAN MATING BEHAVIOR

There is no fundamental difference in the ways of thinking of primitive and civilized man.

— FRANZ BOAS

THOUGHTS ON BEHALF OF A YOUNG WOMAN

Caroline was one of my medical residents. When I knew her, she was twenty-eight, a professional, a wife, and a mother of one child. She was very bright, pretty, and well-educated, yet she struggled with some basic biological decisions. After five years of marriage, she had separated from her husband in what she anticipated would be a temporary arrangement. Only four months later, she found herself falling in love with another man. Having been raised Catholic, she struggled to reconcile her emotions with her religious beliefs. When Caroline brought all this to my attention, we were both busy working in the ER. I had to condense my advice into the following very short historical synopsis.

The Muslim laws of marriage recorded about 700 C.E. were

written by men. Men also wrote the Judeo-Christian marriage laws recorded in the Old Testament 2000 years ago. The earliest known written laws of marriage recorded in the Hammurabi Code 3,700 years ago were written by men. Yet the genetic code that runs Caroline's body and controls her emotions was created millions of years ago and was written by evolution (or, if you prefer, by God). I told Caroline to ask herself why she would allow men to overrule what God had written in her genetic code.

Caroline faces a dilemma that is ubiquitous in modern humans. She is trying to do what she has been taught. However, she has been taught to behave in a way that does not feel right. Each of us has a program written in our genetic code that tells us what feels right, and Caroline has been told that what feels right to her is wrong. She has been taught to act in a manner that contradicts her genetic programming.

Instincts are directed by genetic code. Our bodies and minds follow the instructions recorded in our DNA. As humans became civilized, we learned to act differently for the sake of civilization, but we have deviated so far that we have become confused by our own emotions. We are burdened with guilt and shame for having essentially normal feelings. Guilt and shame destroy our relationships. This could be avoided if we had a better understanding of the origins of our sexual instincts and the modern constraints on our sexual behaviors.

The instincts that drive us today formed in the crucible of the proto-human social environment. They are often in conflict with the modern rules of behavior that developed as we emerged from the Stone Ages a few thousand years ago. How and why did those rules develop? Why do we suppress our instincts? We need to know why we feel one way when we are expected to behave in another.

ORIGINS OF HUMAN SEXUAL INSTINCTS

We will begin by exploring human anatomy and physiology, considering the basic human form and function in the setting of our origins in the early Stone Ages. Most oddities of human sexual behavior result from our walking on two legs, which is not an easy task. Very few animals can do so, and those that can are not able to carry things while walking upright. The great advantage of doing so is that it allows us to use our hands for making tools, carrying materials, and manipulating our environment. However, this combination of traits creates two major engineering problems.

Animals who walk on all fours have the abdominal muscles under their internal organs, providing uninterrupted support. In contrast, a mammal who walks upright must support the abdominal organs on the sling of ligaments and muscles that cross the pelvic opening. That is a challenge because there are openings in the pelvic floor, and organs can push out. A wide pelvic opening causes failures of the pelvic sling, resulting in hernias, uterine prolapse, rectoceles, hemorrhoids, bladder prolapse, and premature deliveries. The pelvic organs protrude out through various openings.

Upright posture also requires the legs and knees to be close together so a person can walk and run without tottering back and forth. (Think of how a raccoon or chimpanzee looks when trying to walk on hind feet.) However, when the knees are close together, it creates a sideways angle between the thigh bone and the leg bone where they meet at the knee. If the pelvis is too wide, that angle is too great, and the kneecap will pop out of place. This is called a patellar subluxation.

Subluxation of the patella is not a big problem nowadays. You just get carried to the local ER to get it fixed. However, if you were being chased by hyenas on the African savannah, it would be a definite game-changer.

. . .

To walk upright and survive, <u>primitive humans needed a narrow pelvis</u>.

Upright posture frees the hands for tasks other than walking. That is the great advantage of bipedalism. We can use our hands to make tools and carry stuff. But freedom for the hands is not enough. It takes a big brain to compete effectively against other proto-humans.

Tool manipulation requires opposable thumbs and highly sensitive hands to recognize the shape of objects by touch. Reach into your pocket and pull out a quarter just by the feel of the coin. This is a rare ability in the animal world. Our fingers can detect the shape of objects in fine detail. We also see in three dimensions with forward-facing eyes and binocular vision. We can discern the shape of objects with our eyes and link it to what we feel with our hands.

It is also not enough to understand only what an object is. To manipulate things, we must have the mental ability to understand what an object can become. Humans can foresee possibilities, consider the future, and compare it to the past. We can visualize what a stone can become if properly worked.

The ability to make a tool from stone does not create a toolmaking culture. Culture cannot develop if each new generation has to rediscover how to break the rocks. The techniques of toolmaking and manipulation of the environment must be taught from one person to another and one generation to the next. This requires memory and language far exceeding those of any other animal.

To make full use of their upright posture, humans needed brains large enough to accommodate tool design, memory, foresight, language, and complex culture. This is problematic because a big brain needs a big head. A human mother must have a wide birth canal to allow the passage of a baby's head.

. . .

In order to birth a baby with a big brain, the human mother <u>needs a wide pelvis.</u>

However, a wide pelvis causes problems when she walks on two legs. It causes uterine prolapse and patellar subluxation. Remember, her pelvic organs need support, and her knees and feet must be close together and under her.

This is called a design conflict. Human females <u>need a narrow pelvis</u> to stand upright, but they <u>need a wide pelvis</u> to birth a baby with a large head. Mother Nature has resolved this dilemma by having human mothers birth babies while the brain is still small, before the head becomes too large. <u>This engineering dilemma is the root cause of all the oddities of human sexual behavior.</u>

Human babies must be born before the brain is fully grown. They are helpless and require a great deal more care than other newborn mammals. Most infant mammals can walk when only a few days old. Some can walk within minutes of birth. It will be two years before a human child can walk reliably without assistance.

The infant's dependency creates a huge burden on the mother. The human mother had to carry and feed her child for about two years. The burden of caring for the child limited the mother's ability to provide for herself and the child. It restricted her ability to move over distances, handle tools, gather food, and brandish weapons. She was at a disadvantage when competing with other humans for food and resources.

It would have been very difficult for a Stone Age single mother to raise an infant alone. She and her child had a greater chance of survival if she had help. The female who could keep a mate at her side, assisting and protecting her and the child, would have had an advantage over females who could not. More of her children would have survived to grow up and have children of their own. But what did the Neolithic female have to offer her mate in return for this devotion? Her assets were very limited.

Fortunately for young women, young men have a critical design trait that makes them easy to manipulate. They are constantly interested in having sex and are incredibly non-selective. Their instincts guide them to do whatever a woman wants in return for sex.

Human males are not like other mammals, which mate only with females who are fertile and able to bear offspring. A buck pursues a doe only during the fall rut. Stallions ignore mares who are not in season. Boars have zero interest in pregnant sows. However, men pursue women regardless of their reproductive status.

Mating behavior is biologically expensive and dangerous. It generates violent conflicts with competing males. It is distracting and exposes an animal to predators. It requires an expenditure of energy in pursuit and mating. It is simply not rational to pursue a female who is not fertile.

Women depend on men being irrational. Human males are genetically programmed to pursue, expend energy on, and give resources to any female who rewards them with sex (or just the possibility of sex). It does not matter that the woman is not ovulating, already pregnant, nursing an infant, past her reproductive age, or simply unavailable.

The other side of this coin is the female's hidden sexual interest. Women need resources throughout the month and all through pregnancy and nursing, so they need the attention of men all the time, not just when they can conceive. For this support system to work, a woman's ability to conceive must be hidden from males. If men were like bucks, stallions, and boars and could tell when a female is ovulating, women would only get what they need from men for a few days every two or three years.

Women do have a genuine interest in sex for its own sake. However, unlike the sustained interest of men, women are highly variable. At any given moment, enough women are interested in sex to keep the men trying, but enough are disinterested to keep men in the dark. Women also change over time, monthly, and throughout life. This variability in desire works well for the human female and her children.

Human sexuality is, above all else, a social support system for mothers of infants and young children. Sex is required to create children, but most human sex serves a different purpose. It aids in the survival of offspring by creating safe environments for the nurturing of children. It is a device women use to obtain child-rearing assistance from men.

Modern Western women often reject this concept. They have been reared in a culture that encourages their independence. They have complete control over their reproductive choices and are taught to support themselves. They have transitioned into adulthood with the confident knowledge that they only have sex when they want to. They do not realize how much their personal sexual freedom is in conflict with the million-year history of humans and with the current status of women in the less-developed world today.

The survival and development of humans required a barter system in which females traded sexual services to men in return for help raising the women's children. Neither the men nor the women knew the role of sex in creating those children. The men knew which women rewarded them with sex. They gave resources and assistance to those women. The women knew which men were helpful and generous providers and used sex to attract those men. Those instincts are still embedded in our subconscious minds, and they are in constant conflict with the rules of modern society.

Unregulated sexual barter is necessarily promiscuous. Men are programmed to give their gametes (sperm) away to any willing female and to purchase the opportunity with resources or labor. Likewise, human females are programmed to trade sex for resources from many males. Sexual promiscuity leads to sperm competition in which a female has semen in her vagina from several males at the same time.

Chimpanzees and the closely related bonobos are highly promiscuous and have a way of dealing with sperm competition.

They have huge testicles and produce a large number of sperm on ejaculation, washing out the sperm of a preceding male from the female's vagina.

Human males have a different way of removing a competitor's semen. They cannot have huge testicles because they walk upright with their testicles between their legs. But they can have a large penis. The diameter of the human penis is much larger than that of any other primate. The tip is rounded, with a flange on the edge of the glans. Experiments have shown these features cause the penis to work like a bilge pump, removing any fluid from a woman's vagina with the first few thrusts of coitus. Small testicles are adaptations to bipedal gait. The shape of the penis is an adaptation to promiscuity.

Standing on two feet frees the hands to manipulate objects, carry things, and make tools. Bipedalism allows for the development of tool-making technology. However, technology cannot advance beyond the primitive level if it must be rediscovered by each new generation. Information must accumulate from one generation to the next, each level building upon the last. This is called hierarchical knowledge. Mother-to-daughter and father-to-son instructions are not sufficient to build a hierarchical knowledge structure. Something more is needed. Any system of technology, even at the Paleolithic level, requires human knowledge reservoirs. Cultural development requires dedicated teachers.

At some time in pre-history, the roles of certain groups changed, probably coinciding with the development of complex language. A fraction of the human population lost reproductive abilities and instead became storehouses of knowledge. This happened in different ways for males and females.

Human females developed menopause, a trait that is unique among primates and very rare among animals. They ceased menses and ovulation after a certain age and stopped having children. Without young children to care for, older women could devote their time to teaching the things they had learned in their lifetimes to their daughters and grandchildren. They became reservoirs of knowledge, more valuable as grandmothers than as mothers.

Males continued to mate throughout their lifetimes, but some did not mate with females. They mated with other males. Free from the burdens of supporting women and children, they had the time to observe where the sun came up each day, build temples to track the seasons, tell people when to plant crops and explore new ways of making tools. They became holy men and priests. These were the men who told the workers where to place the stones at Stonehenge. In the middle bronze age, about 4000 years ago, they introduced the concept of the Sabbath day and created public education. They were the scholars and educators for the community. We will revisit this link between religion and homosexuality in more detail later.

Loss of reproductive capacity is usually detrimental to the survival of a species. However, in an intelligent species with language, homosexuality and menopause paradoxically increased survival by creating intergenerational knowledge reservoirs. The number of offspring was reduced, but the survival of offspring increased enough to offset the losses.

The following list summarizes traits that allow humans to exploit their hands and their upright posture. Among them are some charac-teristically human sexual behaviors, which will be discussed in greater detail later. Consider the roles these attributes may have played in the succession of hominid species that led to Homo sapiens dominance. These are the traits that make us human. They define our sexual instincts and are inescapable.

ATTRIBUTES ASSOCIATED WITH HUMAN UPRIGHT POSTURE

Humans did not develop an upright stance as an isolated trait. To fully exploit this ability, they also needed:

Highly sensitive hands that could grasp and shape objects
Opposable thumbs
Binocular vision and depth perception
Imagination to foresee what an object could become
The ability to sense the shapes of objects by touching them
Language to teach the skills of tool production and use
A brain large enough to perform all these functions
Broad, long, flat feet with short toes
A narrow pelvis to allow upright gait
Early birth before the brain and head are fully grown
A social support system for mothers of helpless infants

- Sustained high sex drive in males
- Highly variable sex drive in females
- Hidden ovulation in females
- Promiscuity
- Homosexual females
- Postmenopausal grandmothers

Small testicles and a large, uniquely shaped penis
Non-reproductive persons to serve as knowledge reservoirs

- Postmenopausal females
- Homosexual males

Bisexual males to propagate the homosexual male genes

HUMAN SEXUAL STRATEGIES

Despite our modern cultures, we are still primitive creatures. Human sexual instincts were formed during prehistory and have not had time to change. Natural human sexuality is very different from what we are taught in modern society. Four concepts are critical to understanding our instincts and their influences.

1. We can choose our behaviors, but we have no choice about our instincts.
2. Primitive humans did not know that sex causes pregnancy.
3. Human sexual behaviors are cultural, but sexual instincts are universal.
4. Men need women, and women need men, but for different reasons.

Reproductive instincts are physiologic responses to stimuli and are not under our control. They are hardwired into the brain and written into the genetic code. Reproductive behaviors, on the other hand, are actions that people choose to take. They are learned from religion, parents, and other cultural sources. Humans can choose their behaviors, but they have no control over their instincts. That is to say, people can control how they behave, but they cannot control how they want to behave.

Behaviors are cultural. They change rapidly with the advancement of history. Think of how clothing styles change yearly. However, reproductive instincts are hardwired into the genetic code and change very slowly. Humans left the Stone Ages a mere ten thousand years ago. They have not had time to change their basic instincts. Humans are still primitive creatures. Men and women, boys and girls, think about each other differently now than they did ten thousand years ago, but they still feel the way they did then. Those two human functions are in constant conflict in our modern lives.

Primitive humans did not understand the relationship between sex and reproduction. They did not know that sex creates babies. This should not be surprising. Male baboons and chimpanzees are not trying to make babies when they copulate with females. They just want sex. The females are not trying to get pregnant. They are just enticing or submitting to the males, depending on where they are in the reproductive cycle.

For primitive humans, reproduction and sex were two unrelated functions. All animals engaged in sex. All female animals birthed young. Primitive humans had no reason to connect the two. They did not discover the link between sex and pregnancy until they domesticated animals. Until then, neither men nor women understood the role of men in creating babies.

It sounds incredulous to us today, but primitive humans did not have the concept of paternity. They did not know that there was a male role in creating a baby. There are indigenous cultures still in existence today who do not understand the male part in conception. Women became pregnant spontaneously or with the help of spirits. They had babies and needed help raising them. Sex was merely a device used by women to get that help.

This explains some important differences between men and women. Since prehistory, mothers have had powerful instincts relating to infants. Prehistoric fathers never developed those instincts. Modern fathers know to attend to their children because they are taught parenting behaviors, but behaviors are different than instincts. A man's instincts tell him that an infant belongs to its mother. When a mother brings a new baby to a public place, other women are drawn to it, but men tend to back away. Men's emotional responses to infants are completely different than women's. When a father engages in parenting of an infant, he is "helping" the mother.

Men have an inclination to nurture and teach children, but it is not instinctively directed to their own children. Primitive men did not have any claim on children. A man had an emotional bond to a woman, but had only an indirect social bond to her children. In most primitive societies, men have no childcare obligations. Fathers' ownership of and responsibilities to children are a modern invention that we will explore later when discussing human families.

. . .

Reproductive instincts must be uniform within a species. That is the definition of a species. The members must be able to breed and create fertile offspring. Two animals with incompatible breeding instincts cannot reproduce. Details as insignificant as single notes in a mating call or the hue of pebbles in a bower can exclude birds from mating. Members of a species must have compatible mating instincts. All humans are in the same species and respond to the same cues. Those cues are programmed in their genes.

Behaviors are a matter of choice. Instincts are not. Dating and marriage customs are behaviors that vary between cultures and religions, but breeding instincts do not. Men and women of all cultures, modern and primitive, have the same stone-age needs and desires. People can choose how they act, but they cannot choose what they want. Their wants are uniform throughout humanity.

Neither a man nor a woman can reproduce alone. This may seem obvious, but it has important implications and needs to be stated. In order for a man to propagate his genes, he must also propagate those of a woman. Likewise, to propagate her genes, she must also propagate those of a man. They become encumbered by each other's genes. It is a mutual burden they cannot escape. However, this was not known by primitive humans any more than it is known by chimpanzees.

The two sexes have different roles and use different strategies in the reproductive process. Men and women have divergent concerns when choosing mates. Like all female mammals, a woman makes a limited number of eggs in her lifetime. She can produce only a small number of children, each of which requires a large investment on her part. She has a womb and breasts. She is the one who bears the greatest share of the burden of nourishing and raising a baby. It is in her best interest, and therefore aids the survival of her genes, to be highly selective in choosing a male to fertilize her ova. Her progeny will need good genes and sustained food and shelter. Her ideal sperm donor would be good-looking, healthy, physically fit, and committed to supporting her and her children. Her instincts direct her to choose men with these traits.

Like all male mammals, a man produces a huge number of sperm and has little investment in them. He can scatter his seed with little consequence to himself. He will have the greatest reproductive success if he impregnates a woman who is good-looking, healthy, and physically fit and has someone, not necessarily him, who is committed to supporting her and her children.

The mother of an infant needs support, but it does not need to be from the biological father of her child. <u>It can be any other man (or men)</u>. In fact, there is no biological reason for her mate to be a man. <u>It can be a woman</u>. Remember, the primitive woman did not know the man's role in creating the child. All she knew was she had a baby, and she needed help.

This is where human sexuality gets so complicated. Human reproductive strategies can range from completely symbiotic, as when a man and woman work together to raise their children, to completely parasitic, as when a woman chooses a different man to be her mate or when a man impregnates a woman and abandons her. They can range from monogamous to polyamorous, with a woman getting support from one or many sexual partners. They can also be heterosexual, as in traditional relationships, or homosexual, as when lesbian couples raise children fathered by men who were transient in their lives. The mother is instinctively bound to her child but not to the child's father. She has many other options in the choice of her mate. A mother's love does not extend to the father of her child. Primitive people did not have the concept of "father of the child." Love is a primitive emotion, not a modern behavior.

Each of us has instincts that serve to propagate our genes – to give our progeny the best chance to populate the planet. You, the reader, are the product of a long line of ancestors who managed to find and retain mates, breed with them, and raise children to adulthood. They did so against astounding odds, outcompeting their adversaries and surviving the hazards of their environments for thousands of generations. You have inherited the genes of millions of winners, and whether you know it or not, you are a savagely competitive creature. Your DNA compels you to compete. Like all humans, you are genetically programmed to cooperate with others, including your own spouse, only when it benefits your progeny.

The idea that men and women compete should not be surprising. The division of labor in human child-rearing places a couple in an adversarial position. Men and women are designed to form reproductive pairs and work together to raise young. However, they both have instincts that drive them to betray their mates.

The human female is genetically programmed to obtain as many resources as possible for her offspring. Therefore, she continues to be sexually active with a man even when she is not fertile or while she is pregnant. She is also inclined to exploit males other than her mate. She knows instinctively that males will offer her incentives in return for suggestions of having sex with her. The shame that modern women associate with this exchange is a learned behavior that will be covered in great detail later.

In modern society, humans are much less promiscuous, and yet women still use their sexuality to obtain social favors. They dress to accentuate their female shape. They wear cosmetics, dye their hair, and have surgery to look younger. Prettier women attract more male attention and obtain more social rewards. They have more opportunities to gain resources. They get more sales to clients and higher tips from customers. Think of the waitresses in bars with low-cut tight blouses and short skirts, flaunting their sexual charms to their customers. Human females still use their sexuality to obtain resources from men because human males still respond to those cues. Those basic instincts have not changed since the Stone Age.

Females with supportive mates have another incentive to stray when they are fertile. Women have different preferences in a male when they are ovulating than at other times. They are genetically programmed to seek out opportunities for sex with males who are more attractive, have more political power, or possess greater wealth than their mates. They may gain additional support and social opportunities, not to mention better-looking children, from such indiscretions.

The human male is inclined to attach himself to a female and support her and her offspring, at least for the time required to raise those offspring through weaning. He benefits from investing resources in the mother of children who are (probably) his progeny. They will be more likely to survive to reproductive age, perpetuating their genes in the gene pool.

However, the human male is also programmed to mate with other females, offering as few resources as possible. Men are inclined to provide resources to any female who promises sex, but they try to minimize their investments in these other females. Primitive men might have offered a freshly caught fish or a piece of honeycomb. Modern men might proffer a one-hundred-dollar bill or a promotion at work.

Men also inflate their desirability. They flaunt or embellish their wealth, choose clothes to accentuate their masculine form and insinuate commitment that is not forthcoming.

An old adage teaches that men court women to obtain sex, while women use sex to get courtship. In human relationships, men want sex, and women want material support. Men need affection, and women need commitment. Men use the promise of commitment to obtain sex, while women advertise their sexuality to obtain resources. Men instinctively want to do nice things for women because there was a time in human development when those efforts were rewarded with sex. Women instinctively desire sex with men who can do nice things for them because there was a time in human history when sex was the commodity women traded for nice things. Are they just using each other? Yes, but that is what they are designed to do. It is all biological, dictated by the anatomy of the knee cap and pelvis.

This crude barter, affection for devotion and sex for support, worked well for primitive people. In today's modern societies, we have rules that govern proper mating behavior. They are dictated by culture, etiquette, law, and religion. However, civilization is only a thin veneer. We are still primitive creatures, and our instincts compel us to behave in an entirely different manner.

This is precisely where my junior colleague Caroline, who I mentioned earlier, finds herself. She is torn between obeying the lessons of her upbringing and answering the call of her instincts. She has been taught that she should remain in love with one man, but she is falling in love with another. To use a computer analogy, her modern software is not compatible with her primitive operating system.

Humans choose new mates quickly when they find themselves alone. In times of personal crisis, natural disaster, or war, the ancient behaviors quickly re-emerge. People revert to their basic instincts. This was well documented in the aftermath of World War II. American soldiers who had money, food, and other resources to spare occupied German cities where local women, many with children, were either widowed or their marital status was uncertain. The German women readily cohabitated with American GIs, the men who may have killed their husbands, to obtain the resources they needed for themselves and their children.

Even the most faithful wife may turn to an alternative man when her children are hungry and her husband's fate is unknown. She will obtain food and protection from any available man and offer affection in return. Men will provide resources to women in return for sex. Allied soldiers fathered 66,000 babies in Germany after World War II. When under stress, humans quickly abandon the idea of monogamy.

MALE AND FEMALE BRAINS

Since the dawn of humanity, there have been distinct differences between the male and female brain. For the most part, both men and women had the same problems to solve on a day-to-day basis: finding food and water, staying warm and dry, and staying out of the claws of predators. Regarding reproduction, though, they had entirely separate, often conflicting, problems to solve. This created important differences between male and female brains, which have not changed since the Stone Age.

Men were faced with a single reproductive problem to solve: how to obtain sex with women. They did not know the role of sex in creating children. They were not trying to beget offspring. They were just in it for the sex. That is why men are so single-minded in pursuit of sex. Their brains are still highly focused on sex. Men have brains that are very task-oriented. They generally think in terms of goals rather than relationships.

Of course, some men were also concerned with power, status, and wealth, but only because it helped them acquire access to women. We still see this today in powerful and wealthy men who put all their achievements at risk by womanizing. Think of Bill Clinton and Jeffery Epstein. Access to women for sex was a higher priority than their political and financial success.

Women, on the other hand, had a completely different problem to solve. They needed to create a safe environment in which to raise their children. This is a nebulous task that requires the ability to work with others. A mother needed to manipulate men in order to obtain the resources and services she needed for child rearing. She also needed to collaborate with other women and create a social structure in her group. She needed to create coalitions of women who would come to her aid against aggressive men. Of course, some women were also concerned with power, status, and wealth, but only to the extent that it secured a safe social environment for their children.

Women's minds are designed for communication and collaboration. They are more empathic and more sensitive to emotions. They are better "mind-readers" than men. They think in terms of social groups and relationships rather than physical structures or isolated tasks.

As Louann Brizendine, MD, says in her two books, *The Male Brain* and *The Female Brain*, men's minds are problem solving machines, while women's minds are communicating machines. The human male mind is designed to achieve specific goals, while the human female mind is designed to generate collaboration and create coalitions.

CHAPTER TWO

NATURAL HUMAN FAMILIES

Sometimes I wonder if men and women really suit each other. Perhaps they should live next door and just visit now and then.

— KATHERINE HEPBURN

In *The Social Organization of Sexuality: Sexual Practices in the United States*, Edward O. Laumann (1994) reports that the average American man would have twelve sexual partners over the course of his life-time, and the average American woman would have six. To some people, this may seem like promiscuous behavior. However, in prim-itive hunter-gatherer societies, men would have had sex at some time in their lives with virtually every adult female in their commu-nity, and most women would have had sex with virtually every adult male. The modern American population studied by Laumann is certainly not monogamous, but "natural" human cultures make modern Americans seem prudish by comparison.

Monogamy is a good example of the conflict between human instincts and contemporary standards of behavior. True monogamy means having only one mate in a lifetime, the fairy tale true love, the one and only soulmate. This is rare in the animal kingdom. There are a few monogamous species, notably swans, snow geese, beavers, bald eagles, prairie voles, and gray wolves. These creatures choose a mate once in adolescence and never do so again. Humans are not like that.

I once had a patient, Mr. Johnston, who came to the ER for chest pain. He was a rancher, and like many independent older men, he was not very adept at talking about his illness. He let his wife answer my questions. During my interview, she disclosed that he started having chest pain when he discovered she was having an affair with one of the ranch hands. In the ER, we know very well that the sinking feeling a person gets in the middle of the chest during emotional trauma can be indistinguishable from the crushing pain of a heart attack. One of the causes of chest pain is a broken heart. Such was the case with Mr. Johnston. He was seventy-two years old, and his wife was seventy-one; yet, she had succumbed to a passionate extra-marital romance and left him with a broken heart.

Human beings retain the capacity to fall in love and to succumb to lust throughout their lives, long past their reproductive years. Humans monitor for alternative mates constantly, even when currently paired. We choose new mates easily throughout our lives, at any age, even long past childbearing age. We typically go through multiple relationships in adolescence before selecting a mate for child-rearing purposes. Once mated, we engage in countless fantasies involving people other than our mates. Some of these fantasies advance to extra-pair couplings, i.e., infidelity. A large number, perhaps a majority, of our long-term, child-rearing relationships end in dissolution. Most of us go on to choose new mates and often remarry. True monogamy is rare among humans. We are not a monogamous species.

I have a colleague and friend named Josh, a very masculine man, one of those men who just drips testosterone. He confided in me once that he did not understand some of his behavior. He has a gorgeous wife who is great in bed and gives him all the sex he wants, yet he is always looking at other women and thinking about approaching them. Josh is under the impression humans are monogamous and men look at other women only when their wives fail to meet their needs. In reality, humans constantly scan for alternative sexual partners, regardless of their current status.

The idea that one man and one woman bond to form a lifelong partnership and "live happily ever after" is a relatively modern invention. The concept linking love and marriage originated in about 900 C.E. in Christian Europe and a bit earlier in the Middle East. Over the preceding 4000 years, marriage in the Middle East and Europe was a contractual arrangement where men owned women. Neither of those arrangements bore any resemblance to primitive natural reproductive relationships.

Under primitive conditions, humans naturally form an astounding array of reproductive arrangements that can be divided into three overlapping categories: polygamous, dioecious, and matrilineal matrilocal. Note that monogamy is not one of them. All three are still present in various parts of the world, including Western societies, where they usually go unrecognized. They are the fallback arrangements when monogamy fails.

In the polygamy model, a person has multiple sexual partners. People often equate polygamy with harems, but harems are rare. They are restricted to a few ostentatiously wealthy and powerful men. Polygamy consists of any person who is regularly sexually active with two or more people simultaneously. Commonly, a man has several women, called polygyny, although one woman can also have several men, called polyandry. Some form of polygamy is still officially sanctioned in about half of the nations on Earth. It also persists unofficially in Western societies, where a wealthy man may have one or more mistresses in addition to his wife, or a woman may have more than one man supporting her in return for affection.

Carl is an executive in a high-paying position requiring frequent travel. He has an ex-wife to whom he pays alimony and child support for two children. He is currently married to his second wife and has one child with her. He also has several mistresses in different towns. I know one of the mistresses. She is married and has a child. The uncertain paternity of the child has been the subject of community gossip. Carl represents the persistence of one of the primitive reproductive strategies. Here is a man who is sexually active with several women on an ongoing basis, a behavior made possible by his wealth and power. He is, for all practical purposes, polygynous.

In the dioecious model, which is Latin for "two houses," the men and women lived in separate physical structures. This family model has had many different labels and variations over the years. It is currently known as sexual segregation. I prefer the botanical term, dioecious. Many indigenous cultures of the Pacific Islands and North and South America lived in this manner before the arrival of Europeans. The women and young children lived in one house, and the men lived in another. When the male children reached reproductive age, they moved to the men's house. Mating occurred between men and women sporadically or in brief relationships. There was no concept of paternity as we know it today.

When I met Deborah, she was twenty-two years old and a single mother who had no contact with the father of her child. She shared a home with three other women, two of whom also had children. They all worked, and some attended college. All the women were heterosexual and dated when they could, often meeting men in bars and occasionally in their work or school.

Deborah illustrates the persistence of the dioecious model for human reproductive behavior. The women and children live in one house. The men live somewhere else. The men and women meet each other out in the world and occasionally mate. Their relationships are sporadic and brief.

Dioecious families can be observed worldwide whenever single women, some with their children, share a home or several men share an apartment. Unwed people generally prefer to share their homes with same-sex peers. It is unusual to find male and female co-habitants sharing sleeping quarters when they are not paired. Segregated college dormitories are officially sanctioned dioecious living arrangements. Even in the now-popular coed dormitories, men and women share the same building but not the same living quarters.

The matrilineal model is the most primitive human family structure. Children identified with and lived with their mothers and grandmothers without knowing their paternal line. In hunter-gatherer cultures, men and women formed pairs, with the man helping the woman raise her children in exchange for her companionship and affection. He may impregnate her, but the children were not recognized as his. Men did not possess children. In the absence of property and inheritance, a male had no incentive to claim children as his own.

In primitive hoe-based agricultural societies, the female was bound to a home and a piece of land. She tended a garden and raised her children, the offspring of different men. Several men would occasionally visit her, bringing gifts in the form of meat or other resources. A man would stay for a while until he tired of the lifestyle or until she tired of him and ran him off. While they were together, they would mate. He would not know his role in the creation of the children. He was just there for the sex. While he was with her, he would indirectly support all the children. After a man left one woman, he went off to stay with another. Soon, another man would appear to take his place.

Catherine is a patient of mine. I have also treated each of her four children, her mother, and her grandmother at various times. She is thirty-two years old and has never been married. She and her children live with her mother and grandmother. The children have three different fathers. All three men are still present, off and on, and occasionally help with groceries. She continues to be sexually active with all three men.

Catherine illustrates the matrilineal model. These three men still provide resources to Catherine and help her raise the children, even though they do not know which, if any, of the children they have fathered. From a reproductive point of view, they are now wasting their time and resources on Catherine because she has had a tubal ligation and cannot produce any more children. Fortunately for her, their basic reproductive instincts are not affected by such trivial matters. Human males provide resources to females in return for sex, regardless of whether the females are fertile.

Catherine's family is matrilineal and matrilocal. The children know who their female ancestors are but not their male ancestors, and they live with their maternal relatives. They identify with their maternal family and have their mother's name. They can be certain of the identity of their mother and grandmother. The identities of their fathers, if known, are much less reliable. The home and children belong to the women. The men are transient in their lives.

Monogamy may be the officially sanctioned family model in much of the world, but it does not occur naturally in humans. Modern humans try to maintain monogamous relationships, but they often fail. When this happens, it is insightful to observe the family models that develop spontaneously. They are polygamous, dioecious, or matrilineal.

CHAPTER THREE

PURPOSE OF ROMANTIC LOVE

Where does the family start? It starts with a man falling in love with a girl.

— SIR WINSTON CHURCHILL

If humans are not monogamous, then why do they fall in love? There are certainly times when they have strongly exclusive relationships, even if only for a short while. Human couples form a special emotional bond called *love*. However, *love* is a nebulous term referring to a wide range of thoughts and feelings. One can love a favorite dress, food, or sport. One loves a spouse, a child, or a pet. People can love their work, country, or God, signifying devotion. All different kinds of love share a common theme. The word *love* can be traced back to the Proto-Indo-European language, and it shares roots with *desire, pleasing,* and *want* in diverse languages, ranging from Sanskrit to German. People can make love, meaning they engage in sex. People can fall into a place or state called *love*. (Also, people can have a score of *love* in tennis, but no one seems to know why.)

Falling in love is somehow different from *love*. It is not the act of loving but rather the act of falling. When one falls in love, there is a sense of collapsing or descending into an emotional condition. There is a feeling of loss of control. For this reason, falling in love is often compared to an illness. A person is referred to as "love-struck" or "lovesick."

In *The Road Less Traveled*, M. Scott Peck constructed a very useful model of the emotional mechanics of falling in love as an ego-boundary process. As a baby grows into a toddler and then into a child, she gradually learns she is separate from the world and the people around her. She develops a sense of what is uniquely her physical self, her space, and her property. She learns she can stop other people from taking things that are hers. She develops a sense of self.

As she grows older, she develops a sense of identity. She recognizes she has a unique personality with her own ideas, desires, plans, wants, and needs. She forms an ego. She also learns about her comfort level with other persons. She discovers, over time, how close she allows other people to be to her, physically and emotionally. She learns how comfortable she is with sharing her space, belongings, and personal information. She develops ego boundaries.

Then, in early adulthood, something happens. This isolated person, wrapped in ego boundaries, meets someone she wants, who also wants her. As they approach each other, their ego boundaries rapidly collapse. They begin to share their wants, desires, and plans. As they grow closer, they share their space and their belongings. What is his is hers. What he wants, she wants. Whatever he wants to do, she wants to do, just to be with him. He will let her into his personal space and share his possessions with her. She will let him into her personal space, let him get close to her, let him touch her body, and even let him inside her body!

Falling in love is a physiological process. A great deal of research is currently being done on the neurochemistry of romance. Two chemicals in the bloodstream and the brain are at the forefront of this research. Oxytocin and dopamine are "feel-good" chemicals. They are associated with relaxation, joy, and contentment. Many other chemicals are involved, too, but their names are irrelevant.

When your lover smiles at you, laughs at a joke, compliments you, or touches your skin, it feels good because your body chemistry has been altered. When your lover kisses or caresses you, the levels of the feel-good chemicals in your bloodstream and your brain rise. This is the reward you receive from a person who puts you at ease because you are attracted to him, and you sense he is attracted to you. The more time you spend with this person, the more you feel at ease and the more easily your body responds to the flood of feel-good chemicals. When you are away from your lover, just thinking of that person causes the release of the chemicals.

In a very short time, this escalates into what could be best described as a catastrophic failure of your personal security system. Your ego boundaries completely collapse. You feel so good with your lover that you care about nothing else. You can think about nothing else. You are love-struck and lovesick.

Love is a grave mental disease.

— PLATO

The two of you have fallen in love. You have merged your ego boundaries, thinking of yourselves as one entity. The two of you have become an "us," a "we." You want nothing except each other. You engage in magical thinking. As long as the two of you have each other, you have everything you need, and you can overcome any hardship. You will climb mountains or swim seas to be together. Love will conquer all. You abandon your families, homes, plans, and common sense to have each other. You cast aside all logic and all precaution, and, without logic or precaution, the two of you mate.

This is, of course, the whole point of it. Falling in love is the process that allows mating to take place. Without it, people would rarely get close enough to each other to have sex. They are too protective of themselves. In the absence of love, people can experience occasional opportunistic sex, violent rape, or other forms of loveless breeding, but they cannot create the sustained sexual activity of lovers that assures pregnancy or the sustained emotional bonds that nurture families. In conceiving and raising young, those couples who fall in love have an advantage over those who do not.

He felt now that he was not simply close to her, but that he did not know where he ended and she began.

— LEO TOLSTOY

CHAPTER FOUR

THE DOWNSIDE: FALLING OUT OF LOVE

Sometimes you have to get to know someone really well to realize you're really strangers.

— MARY TYLER MOORE

Biochemically, falling in love is no different for humans than other mammals. Hormones and chemicals in the brain and bloodstream cause us to relax so much that we allow our lovers to do things we would never tolerate from anyone else. Consider the female cat, who, when in estrus, will let a male approach her, mount her, bite her on the head, and copulate with her. At any other time, she would not let him near her. Of course, the moment they complete the act, she turns and swats at him, indignant that he is in her personal space.

The problem with falling in love is that it does not last. People inevitably fall out of love. Sometimes, it takes years and sometimes a few hours, as in the lyrics of a song describing a woman's morning dilemma. "Whatcha gonna do with that cowboy when he don't saddle up and ride away?" by Chris LeDoux.

In the beginning, falling in love is effortless. It is, after all, falling. Eventually, it starts to require some work. When two people have fallen in love, each tries to be what they think the other wants, but no one can do that for very long. As the novelty of the situation wears off, the level of feel-good chemicals starts to fall. Eventually, the ego boundaries come back, and the two lovers separate. Each starts to protect his own space. Their individual wants and desires re-emerge. She wants to watch TV, but he wants to have sex. He wants to see an action flick, and she wants to watch a chick flick. She wants to redecorate, and he wants to spend the money on a hunting trip. They have become individuals again. The courtship has ended. The honeymoon is over.

Positive emotional experiences dominate new lovers. Their physical bodies are awash in the feel-good chemicals that fuel their desire for each other. However, as they spend time together, they have negative experiences, too. When enough of these accumulate, the actions that once triggered the release of oxytocin cause the release of adrenaline instead, the famed hormone of the "fight or flight response." The lover's touch or the request for attention is no longer pleasurable but becomes an annoyance.

I love being married. It's so great to find that one special person you want to annoy for the rest of your life.

— RITA RUDNER

Love is temporary insanity, curable by marriage.

— AMBROSE BIERCE

Jokes like these thrive in popular culture because we are sympathetic to the characters. We have a certain familiarity with their situations. We all know that the bliss of love fades away in extended relationships. Cynicism in long-term relationships has a valid basis.

Lovers eventually get tired of pleasing each other, and they go back to being individuals with their separate agendas.

Countless song lyrics lament the transience of romance. Think of "April, Come She Will" by Simon and Garfunkel, or "You Don't Bring Me Flowers Anymore" and "Solitary Man" by Neil Diamond. Poetry and lyrics expounding upon the failure of romantic love are popular because they speak to the experiences of almost everyone.

No wonder young people are confused about love. Half of our love songs praise the resilience and permanence of love, while the other half lament love's ephemeral nature and fragility. Our romantic narratives talk of the bliss of never-ending love, while our humor exploits the inevitable demise of devotion. It is all very confusing.

FALSE EXPECTATIONS

> We got married in a fever, hotter than a pepper
> sprout.
> We been talking about Jackson, ever since the fire
> went out.
>
> — BILLY EDD WHEELER AND JERRY LEIBER

Young people go into their relationships thinking they will live happily ever after with their one true love. Then, as love wanes, their feelings get hurt. It is just the ego boundaries coming back up, but that is not how it looks to the two lovers. They have made promises to each other that they cannot keep. Each feels betrayed by the other. Each feels the other either lied about their feelings in the first place or changed their feelings. Of course, they have changed, and they did lie.

It was not malicious lying, but it certainly was misinformation. Women do not lie to their lovers. They "make sacrifices for the sake of the relationship." Men do not lie, either. They call it "courting." However, the truth is she does not like to have sex during primetime TV, and he does not like chick flicks. In fact, each of them did deceive the other.

Now, they find themselves in a relationship that is not following the script they studied. They have read fairy tales, watched romantic films, and studied the dogma of their religion. They have each learned their parts and played them correctly, but they are not living happily ever after. They find themselves fighting an uphill battle against reality, armed only with their unrealistic expectations. Yet, there is nothing wrong with their relationship. It is just following its natural course. The problem is not their relationship but their expectations.

As they gradually become more disillusioned with the relationship, the lovers go through a well-defined progression of stages described by J. Gottman in *Why Marriages Succeed or Fail*. At first, they are content, but as disappointment accumulates, they begin to complain. When that fails to resolve the problem, they advance to criticism. Eventually, they turn to contempt.

Stages of Disillusionment

Contentment:	We're so in love, we don't need to go anywhere.
Complaining:	I wish we could go out to a movie sometime.
Criticizing:	You never take me out anymore.
Contempt:	You never take me out anymore, you cheap bastard.

From Gottman, J. (1995)

Stages of Disillusionment

At the same time, both go through the standard grieving process originally described by Elizabeth Kubler-Ross. They have each lost something important. They have lost that feeling of being in love, that sensation of bliss, that special relationship. They go through the standard grieving process of denial, anger, bargaining, depression, and acceptance. Acceptance is the goal because once that stage is reached, they can get on with their real purpose of raising a family. However, facing dangers along the way, many grieving lovers never reach the stage of acceptance.

The Stages of Grief for Relationships

Denial: "This is just a phase we're going through."
"He's just stressed out about his work (school, parents, health)."
"She's just not feeling well lately."
"We're just taking a time out."

Anger: "I really hate it when he does this."
"She's cut me off just to piss me off."
"I'll be damned if he's getting into my pants anymore."

(This is where some unscrupulous family trial lawyers make their money. They fan the flames of discontent until this natural anger becomes demonic hatred.)

Bargaining: He agrees not to ask for sex until her TV programs are over.
She concedes that he can go hunting.

(This is a genuine attempt by one or both parties to negotiate, offering concessions and voicing their needs. Marriage counselors make their living facilitating this process.)

Depression: The bargaining makes peace, but it does not bring back the lost feelings. Apathy sets in. He drinks too much. She stays in bed all day. They turn to others for sympathy and understanding.

Acceptance: Both parties settle into the realization that the original romance is gone forever. They set aside their feelings and disappointments, accept their situation, and get back to the tasks of raising the kids and running the household.

The Stages of Grief for Relationships

Sadly, both lovers feel they have failed. Their love has not lived up to their expectations. They have "settled" into a lifelong obligation with someone whom they now believe is not their one true love. They do not understand how it happened, and each harbors the grudge that it is the other's fault. They feel shame for what they perceive as their bad choices, guilt for how they have acted toward their partner, and resentment for how they have been treated.

Of course, the fault lies not in the lovers' actions but in their original ignorance about love. They thought they would remain deeply in love, living happily ever after. Wounded by the perceived failure of their relationship and isolated from each other by their hurt feelings, the two lovers do not recognize what they have achieved. Their ego boundaries have reformed, and they are now two separate individuals again. They can now move on to the next level.

THE NEXT LEVEL

Only after two people fall out of love can they start to build a viable long-term relationship. A mature, stable relationship must accommodate the needs of the individuals involved, but before two people fall out of love, they are not acting as separate individuals. Until their ego boundaries reform, they cannot think of themselves as independent persons. They will not express their individual needs. They will make concessions they later regret. They will make promises they cannot keep. An old adage says, "Never believe anything your lover tells you in bed." Until they fall out of love, it is just the hormones talking.

A sustainable long-term relationship must be a co-nurturing process in which the two lovers help each other grow as individuals while working together toward common goals. That cannot happen until they have gone through the ecstasy of ego merging and the agony of ego separation. Enlightened lovers focus on helping each other through this process instead of blaming each other for it. They recognize that relationships change over time and evolve from hormonal to functional. They work together to build a partnership that can survive the challenges of time.

My parents were married for sixty years. My maternal grandparents were married for seventy years, and my paternal grandparents for about the same time. I have countless friends who adore their spouses long after their original romance expired. I have also known countless people who ended up adoring their ex-spouses.

My colleague, John, was a busy physician with a wife and two children. He and his wife had known each other since high school and married young. His marriage was in turmoil to the extent that it often interfered with his work. His wife would come to the office, and they would have loud quarrels. They ultimately divorced, but he stayed close by to help raise the children. Within a year, he was living with her again. They cohabitated for years but never remarried. If they had any further conflict, it was never evident. They stayed together for another decade and finally separated again after the children were old enough to move out. John died after a long illness. His ex-wife cared for him and was at his bedside when he died.

John and his wife got along well after they divorced. Once they had been relieved of the pressure to act as if they were still in love and they accepted that their passion was gone, they were able to get on with their lives. They renewed the friendship they had in their teenage years and attended to the tasks of raising their children and taking care of each other.

THE POST-ROMANTIC RELATIONSHIP

A complex, costly behavior pattern such as monogamy cannot persist in a population unless it offers some survival advantage. Monogamy persists in human societies because extended child nurturing by two parents is beneficial. People try to be monogamous because it is the best way to raise healthy, well-educated children in modern technological culture. Likewise, civic leaders try to convince people to be monogamous to benefit those civilizations.

Sustained long-term relationships are necessary today simply because the structure of human society is so different now than it was ten thousand years ago. Primitive family structures were good enough for humans when life was primitive. The population density was lower. People did not move frequently. They lived in villages surrounded by extended family. Most of a child's education came from other members of the village. The body of human knowledge was small and could be learned by casual association.

Today's children are not immersed in a village of intimate friends and relatives. In all but the most rural places on Earth, children today are surrounded by strangers. Their rearing depends on a strong nuclear family unit. Culture has advanced to the point that each person owns only a tiny fraction of the body of human knowledge. Informal education cannot provide for the needs of modern children. It now takes eighteen years or more to teach children what they need to know.

We now return to the question I asked my junior colleague Caroline. Why would she allow men to overrule the instructions given to her through her genetic code? It is because she lives in a modern world. She does not live in a primitive society. She believes her son will thrive better in a two-parent patriarchal household. She believes this because it has been taught to her by her parents, society, and culture. Her religion has also taught her that a woman's natural role is to be subservient to one man throughout her lifetime. This, however, does not feel right to her, and she does not understand why.

It is not natural for humans to form lifelong, monogamous relationships any more than it is for humans to take medicines or sit for long hours in classrooms. Lovers should know in advance that monogamy is an artificial behavior. It is a worthy goal and has a valid purpose, but it is difficult and uncomfortable for humans. Couples who understand this can avoid the feelings of shame, guilt, and resentment that destroy an intimate relationship. When falling out of love results in hurt feelings, all the joy is driven out of the relationship. If lovers understand that falling out of love is part of the natural progression in a relationship, they have a much better chance of retaining their original intimacy as they graduate into a mature, nurturing partnership.

Making the post-romantic transition is tough. A mature partnership is a completely different emotional arrangement than the bond shared by a couple who have only recently fallen in love. It is held together by an entirely different set of instinctive behaviors that have little to do with romance. When applied to post-romantic relationships, the word *love* has little to do with passion. The expression "I love you" ceases to mean "I have the hots for you" and instead means "I want to reassure you that I still plan to be your social partner for the long term." Although passion and intimacy may have their place, the couples who succeed in constructing durable long-term relationships will be those who recognize the value of good friendship and the golden rule.

CHAPTER FIVE

PAIR BONDS

Love is only a dirty trick played on us to achieve continuation of the species.

— W. SOMERSET MAUGHAM

Falling in love is not without costs. It is emotionally, socially, and economically expensive. Both members of a pair put their resources and reputations at risk. Yet it is short-lived. In *Anatomy of Love,* Helen Fisher, Ph.D., an anthropologist at Rutgers University, wrote that falling in love is like the seasonal pair-bonding in birds and other animals. It lasts only for a set period required to raise a brood. Humans can reproduce without pair bonds, but the pair bond performs several important functions.

Many people use *serial monogamy* to describe human relationships, but it is a poor substitute for *pair bonding*. It implies human relationships are naturally sexually exclusive. They are not. The situation is much more complex than that. Virtually all modern societies encourage people to enter lifelong marital arrangements that include an obligation to fidelity. There are good reasons for doing so, but many people fail to adhere to those rules. They are plagued by temptation because they are naturally inclined to have both romantic and sexual interactions with people other than their mates. Humans are simply not monogamous by nature.

Pair-bonding is a more accurate descriptive term for the natural form of human reproductive relationships. This means two individuals join to raise a brood of offspring cooperatively. The pair bond lasts for the length of one breeding cycle. Most birds, a few mammals, and even a few fish do this, but birds are the best example. The male and female join for a single season to mate, build a nest, hatch the eggs, and nurture the young.

For centuries, nesting birds have been admired as models of fidelity. Under the scrutiny of modern science, though, they have fallen from grace. Virtually every one of the passerine (perching) birds studied thus far – and these comprise more than half of all bird species – turn out to be unfaithful to their mates to some degree. Careful DNA analysis of the droppings from under nests shows that up to forty percent of chicks are not the offspring of the male who helped raise them. Furthermore, with rare exceptions, pairs of birds separate after the brood is raised and never see each other again. Even among the most faithful species, such as mourning doves, a pair will separate and abandon the nest they have built if they do not produce an egg in a timely fashion.

The work by Helen Fisher provides a compelling argument that Homo sapiens is a pair-bonding species. Her transcultural studies of divorce rates demonstrate a peak at four to seven years of marriage. Under natural conditions, the human male and female form a union lasting that long, allowing the rearing of one or two children through weaning. The couple then separates, and each spouse finds other mates and raises additional families. Each adult typically forms four or five such unions throughout a lifetime. This pattern persists unrecognized in modern societies around the world. More than half of marriages end in divorce, and most divorced people remarry. Subsequent marriages have higher divorce rates than first marriages.

One would expect human beings to become better at a task with practice. If they are monogamous by nature and try to be monogamous in their relationships, then divorce rates should fall in subsequent marriages. This is not the case. First marriages have a fifty-percent divorce rate. Most of these divorcees will remarry, and the divorce rate for second marriages is seventy percent. The divorce rate for third marriages is eighty percent. Practice does not make people better at being married. Rather, it seems to make them better at divorcing. Perhaps they simply become more adept at recognizing when to quit a relationship that has exhausted the pair bond. However, the result is that no matter how hard they try to be monogamous, most humans end up with a life history of a series of pair bonds.

In most primitive cultures, both males and females are free to engage in extra-pair couplings while pair bonded. Many primitive cultures encourage both parties to have multiple partners. Despite sanctions against extramarital sex and strict penalties for infidelity, promiscuity persists in the modern world. Fifty percent of women and seventy percent of men are unfaithful. Modern humans are thus no more inclined than their primitive ancestors to have exclusive sexual relationships. From the dawn of history, they have habitually sought sexual partners outside of their primary unions. It is basic human nature.

Why do fools fall in love? Why do they fall in love?

— FRANKIE LYMON

What, then, is the point of the pair bond? Humans have evolved (or are designed) to fall in love. They go through all the trouble of forming a special relationship with one individual of the opposite sex only to cheat on that person and eventually separate. If the pair bond is transient and non-exclusive, what adaptive purpose does it serve? Why don't people just choose mates on an intellectual, political, economic, or random basis? Well, many cultures do just that. They arrange marriages without any input from the two parties bound by the arrangement. Intriguingly, their divorce rates are much lower than those in Western cultures. So why do people fall in love?

Perhaps falling in love is a reliable way to choose the best mate for lifelong love, support, and the rearing of children, but this is doubtful. People fall in love with the most inappropriate persons. They fall in love with people who are already pair-bonded or are incapable of bonding. They fall in love with persons who could never possibly raise or support a family, people who are grossly irresponsible, chronically destitute, or in prison. Women fall in love with men who killed their previous wives, and men fall in love with women who demonize their three previous husbands. Men fall in love with men, and women fall in love with women. Falling in love is far from infallible as a method of choosing the perfect mate for rearing a family.

Perhaps falling in love serves to identify a mate appropriate for a person's social network, but the evidence is to the contrary. It may do just the opposite. People fall in love with others who are totally at odds with their social network. They often search outside their local social circle for mates. They find themselves in love with persons of different races, religions, social backgrounds, and ages, or people who are completely unacceptable to their parents and families. The classic love stories share a common theme of impossible love between members of different social classes, as in *Cinderella*, or warring factions, as in *Romeo and Juliet*.

Perhaps falling in love guarantees one will live "happily ever after." Again, the evidence argues against it. The pair bond is a short-lived phenomenon. People fall out of love. The honeymoon ends. Fairy tales are filled with couples who live their lives together in bliss from their first kiss in adolescence, but in real life, the bookstore shelves are filled with volumes advising people on how to struggle through marriage after the honeymoon ends.

Why do humans fall in love and form pair bonds as their

preferred mating strategy? This must somehow be adaptive. It must provide some advantage to the lovers and their progeny, or the behavior would not persist. People would not be made this way unless it served some purpose.

Humans can reproduce without falling in love, but the pair bond expedites and fine-tunes mating in several important ways that aid in human survival. First, it allows two persons to be lovers and to create offspring. That is, it allows their ego boundaries to collapse so the two separate individuals, each with their own personal space, can trust each other enough and get close enough to become lovers. It expedites mating and the mixing of gametes, the joining of sperm and ovum.

Of course, women can get pregnant without falling in love. There are hundreds of other reasons for having sex besides being in love, and all of them can result in pregnancy. However, most pregnancies result from two persons knowing and trusting each other well enough to merge their personal spaces, remove their clothing, make bodily contact, and lose themselves in the passion of loving until their gametes mix. This requires the level of trust that comes with pair-bonding.

The pair bond helps humans care for babies, just as it does for many animals with extremely infantile, dependent offspring. Pregnancy and nursing burden the human female, limiting her ability to provide for herself and her children. She is dependent on a mate to help her until her children can walk and feed themselves. Female human ancestors who could attract and hold a partner's devotion had more resources to care for their babies. They had more food, shelter, and protection compared to a single mother, and more of their offspring survived. The same is true of the males who stayed with their mates and helped raise their young. Their children had a higher survival rate compared to the offspring of non-pair-bonding males.

Finally, pair-bonding restricts humans to relatively unfamiliar persons in their choices of mates. Paradoxically, humans rarely fall into romantic love with people they already know well. This is called the Westermarck effect, after the man who first noted that people who are raised as children in the same household do not fall in love as adults, even if they are unrelated. This has been confirmed repeatedly, especially in the setting of communes in the second half of the 1900s, where children raised communally rarely chose marriage partners from their communes.

Humans cannot drop their ego boundaries and merge with other individuals they know too well. There must be some mystery about a person for a love interest to occur. Perhaps people who know each other well cannot deceive themselves into overlooking each other's faults or cannot hide their intentions and desires. Love is blind, and apparently, blindness is a prerequisite for love. It is physically possible for a brother and sister to engage in sex, but they are not inclined to do so. Their ego boundaries prevent it. They cannot get that close without being offended by each other's presence in their personal space. They cannot fall into romantic love. The pair-bonding process inhibits incestuous romance.

For the same reason, pair-bonding reduces population inbreeding and promotes genetic mixing. In primitive tribal societies, pair-bonding causes adolescents to move from one clan to another. They are more inclined to choose a mate from outside their family circle and friends than from within. Girls are more interested in boys from the next village than the boys with whom they grew up. Of course, the corollary to this is familiarity breeds contempt: after people get to know each other too well, they fall out of love. The period of blissful ignorance expires. The pair bond starts to dissolve.

Unlike birds, modern human children do not leave the nest at the end of the pair bond. The endpoint of the relationship in humans is not clear-cut. Instead, the couples are bound together financially but drift apart emotionally. They lose interest in each other, get annoyed with each other, and start looking at alternatives. That is, they begin to stray.

REPRODUCTIVE STRATEGIES

David Buss and David Schmitt from the University of Michigan Department of Psychology have described human mating strategies and the inclination to cheat. Their model divides human mating behavior into short-term and long-term strategies separately for males and females. Each of these four strategies has certain problems to be solved, rules to be followed, rewards to be gained, and risks to be incurred.

Pair-bonding is the core of the long-term strategy for both males and females, but the sexes are genetically programmed to have divergent concerns when choosing a long-term partner. Males and females judge potential mates according to different criteria, reflecting their opposing needs.

The female has a relatively small number of opportunities for reproduction in her lifetime, and each of her offspring will require a large investment on her part. She will have greater reproductive success in the long run if she is very selective. She seeks the greatest amount of commitment and support and the highest quality genetic material, but the support and the genetic material do not have to come from the same person.

The human female tries to pair bond with a long-term mate based on emotional commitment and wealth more than on attractiveness. She must locate and attract a man who has resources that will persist over some time, long enough for her to raise a child. He must be willing to bond with her and commit those resources to her and her offspring. Also, she would prefer that he have good-quality genes, which she will judge by his attractiveness.

However, the attractiveness of the long-term mate is not of great importance to a woman. She can pair bond with a good provider and then utilize extra-pair couplings to obtain genetic material for her offspring. That is, she can cheat on her partner by having a more attractive lover on the side. If she is willing to take risks, a woman can have the best of both worlds. She can pair bond with a male who has the resources to commit to her offspring and still combine her genes with those of a more attractive male who is not willing to support her.

Human females have other reasons for seeking short-term mates. They may gain resources and increased social status in return for sex. Sexuality is a tool women use to obtain resources and social favors from men.

A male searching for a long-term mate looks for a female who is able to reproduce but is not already pregnant. He desires a woman with prominent breasts, a narrow waist, and full hips and buttocks. Youth and an hourglass figure are the epitome of female beauty. She should not be overly burdened with children from previous mating. He wants some of her time for himself. She should possess good genetic material, which he will judge by her attractiveness.

She must be obtainable. She must be willing to submit to him in return for the resources and commitment he can offer so that he is not wasting his time. That is to say, she has to want him too. Men searching for a long-term mate are unlikely to pursue women with higher social status or earning power than themselves.

In contrast, a male searching for short-term mating opportunities is very non-selective. He has an endless supply of gametes to put wherever he has the opportunity, with potentially no further investment on his part. He enhances his reproductive success by forming a pair bond and supporting the mother of his children, but he has other options.

Human males are genetically programmed to spread their seed wherever they can. When men search for opportunistic mating partners, the main emphasis is on availability, while attractiveness is less important. The pair-bonded male who seeks additional females does so with no intention of making any investment in the female beyond some honeycomb, a fresh-caught fish, a bottle of wine, a nice meal, or a one-hundred-dollar bill. He trades resources for an opportunistic coupling, and then he is gone. He has lots of gametes to spare and very low biological risk.

A gallivanting male would prefer short-term mating with a highly attractive female if one were available. The offspring of a promiscuous male would benefit most if he impregnates a female who is pair-bonded to a man with resources. The children would be raised well and fare better than if the female were unsupported. However, such a woman is likely to require more of his resources and time before she submits. This costs him more, and it puts him at another risk. The more time he is away from his mate, the more opportunity she has to stray or to entertain other men.

When one man impregnates another man's wife, the traditional name for this is "cuckolding," after a family of birds, the cuckoos, who lay their eggs in the nests of other birds. The cuckoo egg hatches earlier than the host's eggs, and the cuckoo chick pushes the rightful eggs out of the nest. The nest owners do not recognize that the sole remaining chick in the nest is not their species, and they feed it until it grows to maturity and flies away to parasitize some other hapless couple.

Cuckoldry happens commonly in humans. With modern blood typing, tissue typing, and DNA sequencing techniques, paternity is no longer a mystery. It has become a simple matter to determine whether the father of a woman's child is, in fact, her husband. Depending on the academic study and the demographic group, one to thirty percent (average four percent) of children born to married women are the product of extra-pair couplings. For one out of 25 children, the genetic father is not the woman's husband, a condition known as paternal discrepancy. This should not be surprising. Both men and women are inclined to engage in infidelity.

Cuckoldry is a viable reproductive strategy, but not without risks. The gallivanting male may be discovered if the mate of his chosen lover is practicing competent mate-guarding. Jealousy over mates has always been one of the most common causes of homicide among human males. Even today, some states in the U.S. allow a "crime of passion" defense. That is, the courts will excuse a man for killing another man he finds with his wife.

In primitive societies, such as the Kalahari Bushmen of southern Africa, the homicide rate among males is thirty percent. That is to say, three out of ten adult males die from homicide. The most common cause is jealousy. Mating can be a dangerous game.

A few years ago, a fifty-year-old married attorney, the father of three adult children, came to me with facial injuries, including a broken nose, after being assaulted by the husband of his mistress. She was forty and the mother of two grown children, but she was very pretty and looked much younger. She was a paralegal working for the attorney. They had been having an affair that was well-known in the community. Her husband worked out of town on alternate weeks, which gave her ample free time. Eventually, the husband discovered the affair and went to the attorney's office, where the two of them had a verbal confrontation that escalated into a fistfight. The attorney lost.

Even today, among civilized, well-educated men, jealousy over women is a common cause of violence. Every human male has the instinct to kill a rival over a sexual partner. In less civilized times and places, this confrontation might well have ended in murder.

The risk-benefit ratio for infidelity is completely different for males and females and dictates different behaviors for optimal survival. When conceiving her offspring, the female benefits from mixing higher-quality genetic material with her own. She may also receive pleasure, resources, food, social status, or opportunities. She is genetically programmed to accept lovers who either offer resources or are more attractive than her long-term mate. The benefits she gains from extra-pair couplings will be social. She does not get additional offspring or any increase in the propagation of her genes. She is generally limited to one pregnancy every two years, no matter how much she copulates. She also risks offending her current pair-bonded mate and losing her source of support if he questions her devotion or the paternity of her offspring. This is why women who stray tend to be selective and discreet.

The human male has the potential to benefit biologically from every extra-pair coupling. Every tryst may result in additional offspring, another copy of the male's genes in the gene pool, requiring no further investment on his part. Males are inclined to be less discerning than females. This is not because they foresee the value of additional offspring but rather because males with this characteristic have historically had more children. Thus, most men are now hardwired to couple with any female, regardless of her attractiveness, if she is interested. Men may prefer chastity in long-term mates, but they want a short-term mate to be easy. Their only risks are loss of the resources they expend and any personal dangers they incur. They will be discreet only when required to protect their safety. If a man is highly attractive, he may benefit from advertising his availability because pair-bonded females with less attractive mates will seek him out. Some musicians and professional sports figures are notorious for this.

To summarize, both male and female humans are genetically programmed to form pair bonds as their long-term mating strategy. A male looks to pair bond with a healthy, attractive female capable of raising children. A female looks for a healthy, wealthy male capable of protecting and providing for her and her children.

Both males and females are genetically programmed to seek short-term mating opportunities outside their pair bond. Males are programmed to take advantage of any opportunity to copulate with any available female. Females are programmed to engage in extra-pair couplings discreetly and selectively only with males who are more attractive than their current mate or who offer resources or opportunities in return for sex. This is the core of human reproductive strategies. Everything else is just variations on this theme.

HISTORICAL NOTE

A physician named Cecil Jacobson, who ran a fertility clinic in Washington, D.C., in the 1970s, is the master of human cuckoldry. His practice included artificially inseminating women who were married to infertile men. His services were not covered by medical insurance, and his clients were all wealthy enough to pay out of pocket. Dr. Jacobson told his clients that he used semen from a local sperm bank. However, the enterprising doctor reduced his overhead costs by using his own semen. By the time one of the couples noticed that their child resembled the doctor, he had successfully treated the infertility of seventy-five couples. Dr. Jacobson committed an astounding array of ethical and legal offenses for which he was incarcerated. Nonetheless, he enjoyed tremendous reproductive success. He fathered seventy-five offspring, all of whom were raised by affluent pair-bonded couples.

CHAPTER SIX

WHAT IS ATTRACTIVE?

Mr. Winwood Reade, however, who has had ample opportunities for observation, not only with the negroes of the West Coast of Africa but with those of the interior who have never associated with Europeans, is convinced that their ideas of beauty are ON THE WHOLE the same as ours.

— CHARLES DARWIN, *THE DESCENT OF MAN*

What do people look for in a mate? To both sexes, attractive means physical beauty, symmetry of facial features, good posture, clear skin, healthy hair, absence of physical deformities, and other evidence of good general health. It also includes the absence of foul odors and dispositions. A nice smile, a pleasant voice, and a cheerful mood are important to men and women. No one likes someone who is blatantly offensive in his or her appearance, odor, or personality. Beyond that, both males and females are hard-wired to like certain things in a mate.

WHAT DO MEN WANT?

A human male is designed to prefer certain physical characteristics in a female. Breasts are necessary for nursing offspring and are physical evidence of the female's ability to care for infants. Likewise, wide hips are evidence of the female's ability to deliver babies and survive childbirth. Smooth body contours are evidence of her state of nutrition. Healthy women have a layer of fat under their skin, representing a storehouse of food, which they will mobilize to produce milk for their offspring. This layer of fat gives them their feminine curves instead of the muscular sculpturing of men.

The human male also prefers a female with a narrow waist. This may seem paradoxical because it limits a man's choices to women with relatively low body fat, but the narrow waist excludes most women who are already pregnant. A reproductively successful male does not expend his time, resources, and gametes on a female who is pregnant by someone else. This is not for any cognitive reason. Basic instincts do not rely on intellect. Men do not understand why they have these desires. It is simply because men with such preferences propagated more of their genes than men who did not; thus, most men now have those predilections. Men favor women with a waist-hip ratio of 7:10, whether in the African bush, the southern tip of South America, the Asian Steppes, the Australian Outback, or New York City. Men on all continents and in all cultures and races prefer women with an hourglass figure.

Men also instinctively seek young women. When a man impregnates a woman, he procures her services to care for his progeny and propagate his genes for the rest of her life. A younger female has more years available to dedicate to his offspring. A younger woman has more reproductive value than an older woman because she has a greater life expectancy. Human males universally equate youth with beauty.

This explains why women work so hard to improve their physical appearance. They select clothing that accentuates their female form.

They wear makeup and dye their hair to hide their age and to look more healthy and youthful. It increases their ability to use sexuality to influence men. It also explains why some extremely patriarchal cultures force women to hide their bodies. It disempowers women, preventing them from using sexuality to influence and exploit men.

In the selection process, some females are left out. Ultimately, in humans (and all animals that copulate), males choose their female mates, and male preferences determine female characteristics. The opposite is also true. Females choose males to mate with, and some males get left out. Females determine male characteristics. This is the natural order of things, which Darwin called sexual selection. Whether by chance or design, it is the way nature is supposed to work. Survival of the fittest is sometimes the same as survival of the prettiest.

WHAT DO WOMEN WANT?

Women also look for certain physical characteristics. A woman instinctively prefers a man who can protect her and her offspring. She is attracted to a man with good muscle mass, above-average height, and an athletic physique. A light step, quick movements, and coordination are desirable. Women like men who can dance or who succeed in sports.

However, women's likes are more complicated than that. The peacock is a standard model for male attractiveness. A peacock attracts the attention of the peahens by displaying huge, brilliant tail feathers. Such tails would seem to be detrimental to their owners. They have no intrinsic survival value at all. The tails are large, bulky, and highly visible to predators. They are a hindrance to a peacock who needs to forage in difficult terrain or escape a predator. They also require a huge investment of dietary protein and other nutrients.

The peacock strategy is common among vertebrates. The male is communicating to the peahen that he has resources to waste. He is providing her with visible evidence that his genes and his ability to find food and escape predators are so good that he can display this ostentatious tail and get away with it. The tail is an example of bravado, showing off the quality of one's genes.

As a sexual strategy, it works. The female buys it. She does so because it is a valid representation of the quality of the male's genes. He must be an exceptional survivor to produce and maintain such a tail. It is in her best interests to have those genes for her offspring. It is in the best interest of her sons to have tails like that so they will be able to attract peahens and carry her genes into the next generation. She is genetically programmed to choose the guy who is the biggest showoff. It is survival of the prettiest.

David is a colleague of mine. He is a tall, good-looking professional who drives a brightly colored sports car. He has been married and divorced twice and pays child support to four different women. His first live-in girlfriend had a set of twins before they separated. His first wife had a single child by him. His second wife had two children, and his latest girlfriend has a single child with him.

David is like the peacock with the brightest tail feathers. Women flock to him because of his good looks, high earning power, and expensive car. He has had good reproductive success. He probably has additional offspring he is not supporting. There is a high likelihood he has cuckolded other men. He has the genetic material women look for when they roam.

Men are like peacocks in their own way. In primitive societies, they wear the brightest bird feathers they can find or dive from trees with vines tied around their ankles. In our culture, they drive oversized pickup trucks or sports cars. They engage in rowdy, dangerous behavior, make loud music, cover themselves with tattoos, and play rough games. Race car drivers, bull riders, rock musicians, and professional athletes all have their groupies.

Theresa was a forty-two-year-old married professional woman visiting from out of town for a conference when she gave in to her primitive short-term mating instincts. She sought an attractive lover for a one-night stand while away from her husband and social network. Unfortunately, things went wrong when the condom slipped off his penis, placing her at risk of both pregnancy and discovery. She arrived in my ER just after midnight in a panic, asking us to remove the condom from her vagina and to prescribe a "morning-after" pill. She was in the company of an embarrassed twenty-year-old local cowboy who was her partner in this short-term mating adventure. She was available, and he had no reason not to engage in sex with her. However, he did incur some risk. He was embarrassed by the incident, being identified as the male whose penis was too small for the condom.

When searching for short-term mating opportunities, human females seek out males who advertise the quality of their genes through their expensive toys and dangerous behavior. This is why men do such foolish things. They ride bulls, race cars, ride motorcycles, smoke cigarettes, disregard authority, and jump off cliffs into shallow water. They do it to impress women, which apparently works. This is why good girls like bad boys. Rowdy boys are showing off their good genes. They have energy and resources to waste. That is why they are so interesting and entertaining, unlike a man who is merely a good, stable provider.

Eric came to my ER with a broken ankle. He was with a group of college students on a canoeing trip. They stopped in an area of the river with cliffs lining one shore. The girls were swimming in the water and sunbathing on the opposite shore while the boys were jumping into the water from successively higher cliffs. They kept at it until Eric broke his ankle and had to be taken to the hospital.

This is typical bravado. Boys show off. They do so partly to get the attention of the girls, but even if the girls were not watching, the boys were watching each other. They were engaged in a competition to determine who could be the most reckless without getting injured. Eric lost.

Often, men are trying to impress other men. They know the advantages of a man who stands out in the crowd and is admired and respected by other men. Women are aware that men know which males have the best survival potential. They are attracted to leaders and men with political power. Power is universally attractive to women. The captain of the football team is more tempting than one of the linemen. The CEO of a corporation is a better catch than one of the salesmen. The village headman is more attractive than the village cobbler.

Power is the ultimate aphrodisiac.

— HENRY KISSINGER

The attractiveness of rowdy boys and powerful men is why women sometimes do such foolish things, like having an affair with their husband's boss or with their married gynecologist. This is why a twenty-year-old White House intern sneaks into a closet with a sixty-year-old man for clandestine sex.

This is also why a woman will sometimes yield more easily to a proposition from an irresponsible man than to a solicitation from a quality male who has the potential to be a long-term mate. She sees the former as a short-term mate only and acts accordingly. However, when a quality man approaches, she will display chastity and play hard to get, trying to exhibit the qualities of a good long-term mate.

Likewise, a man may spend excessive money on a woman of poor mate potential, anticipating immediate rather than long-term rewards. The same man may behave more frugally and responsibly around a woman whom he wishes to woo as the mother of his children. Women know this, and those who consider themselves a long-term investment may refuse excessive gifts. They are communicating that they want a monogamous relationship rather than a fling.

However, monogamy has its costs.

CHAPTER SEVEN

THE MONOGAMY DILEMMA

All who have meditated on the art of governing mankind have been convinced that the fate of empires depends on the education of youth.

— ARISTOTLE

Humans are not naturally monogamous, and yet we try to convince ourselves we are. We have good reasons to do so. The behavior provides advantages to the individuals who practice it. Cultures that encourage monogamy are more likely to survive than promiscuous cultures. However, monogamy has costs in terms of lost opportunities, personal loneliness, and efforts to keep human instincts in check.

Our natural reproductive behaviors served us well until a few millennia ago. Under primitive conditions, parents raised their children only through weaning. After that, the tribe or village raised the children. The parents separated to find new mates and make more babies.

This is exactly where my junior colleague Caroline finds herself.

She and the father of her child have fallen out of love, and she is searching for a new mate. She is following her genetic programming, doing what feels right to her, even though it violates the rules of her culture. She was taught that she and her husband would stay in love, but her emotions have followed an entirely different course – one that is more consistent with human nature.

While human genetics have changed very little during the past 10,000 years, the social structure of humanity has changed enormously. We are still inclined to pair bond, but the pair bond interval is far too short for the educational needs of the modern world. Technological cultures require extended parenting and education. Any culture that can keep parents together beyond the natural pair-bond duration will have an advantage over those that do not. A few short years of dual parenting may be adequate to assure the survival of the children of Kalahari Bushmen, but it is not enough time to educate citizens of the modern world. This is part of the answer to the question I offered to Caroline. She feels compelled to ignore her instincts and follow the rules of society because she knows a two-parent upbringing is best for her child and best for the society and culture in which she lives.

Under natural conditions, children drift away from their parents' control shortly after weaning and are raised by the general community. Their education is informal, coming from older relatives in the village, and continues throughout their lives. They become adults and begin sexual activity when they reach puberty. This is the social environment in which early humans, our Paleolithic ancestors, thrived. People in primitive societies still live this way.

As cultures compete for land and resources in an overpopulated world, some survive, and some perish. The survival of advanced societies is utterly dependent on investment in many years of childhood education. The society that does the best job of educating its youth dominates other societies economically and militarily. By extension, the society that keeps parents together to raise their children through college has the advantage over those in which parents raise their children only through kindergarten. The chances of survival are enhanced for both progeny and culture when parents remain devoted to each other and raise their children beyond the natural duration of their pair bond. Ultimately, the most successful culture is the one that best persuades parents to stay together "for the sake of the children." All measures of childhood achievement show the best parenting is long-term dual parenting. Nevertheless, long-term parenting is not without problems.

The extended parenting of modern civilizations requires children to remain under their parents' supervision and control long past early childhood. Parents tightly control contact with other adults and children. Children are sent to schools, confined on campuses, and made to adhere to artificial schedules. Contact with their peers is rigidly restricted to non-sexual activities. This is all very unnatural and does not seem fair to adolescents. It does not feel right to them, and, not surprisingly, they resent it. That is why many teenagers are so rebellious, and the strong-handed support of authorities is often required to ensure compliance. It is also why some children completely reject the control of their parents, either by engaging in contrarian behavior or by running away. Humans are not yet a fully domesticated species.

Adolescents have powerful hormonal drives to leave their parents and find mates of their own. In our modern societies, the restrictions they live under feel wrong and unjust. Human adolescents are not designed to stay at home as long as they do. The conflict between adolescents and adults has historically inspired young adults to advance the spread of humanity around the globe by leaving home.

As is often the case, what is difficult for children is even more difficult for their parents. Consider the strain of extended child-rearing on the parents, who are well equipped emotionally to raise small children but are at a loss for skills to control adolescents. The conflict between children and parents in homes with teenagers is trans-cultural. It is a staple theme in literature in all cultures.

The conflict between children and adults in extended pair bonds is minor compared to the conflict between adult parents. The original pair bond is held together by selflessness that comes from the collapse of ego boundaries and the merging of egos. Once those ego boundaries re-form, couples are no longer lovers but ex-lovers. They find themselves obligated for life to a home, mortgage, family, and marriage with a relative stranger whom they may or may not like. Keeping them together as faithful couples is a tough task.

Monogamy may be best for children and society, but it is not what humans are designed to do. It is uncomfortable for humans to extend the pair bond beyond its natural length. As the bond wanes, couples cease loving each other and often cease liking each other as well. Their mutual lust vanishes. The woman tires of having sex with a man she doesn't like, and the man tires of paying bills for a woman he doesn't like. No matter how strong their genuine friendship used to be, they eventually become embittered about their relationship, not understanding how it came to be this way. They do not understand that this is the natural course of a relationship because they do not understand the nature of the original pair bond. Such embitterment ruins relationships between people who often started as good friends. They accumulate anger and resentment, which interferes with their companionship.

Perhaps this is the reason many couples become better friends after a divorce. In *The Good Divorce*, Constance Ahrons wrote that about fifteen percent of divorced couples return to being good friends. Another thirty-five percent remain on relatively good terms and co-parent their children with minimal conflict. Her studies show that half of the divorced couples get along better after the divorce than before. Once they abandon the unrealistic expectations associated with the original pair bond, they can go back to being friends again.

After a pair bond expires, a married couple remains dependent on each other to meet their emotional, economic, personal, and sexual needs. They are forbidden from seeking solace outside the marriage. Each becomes increasingly disinterested in meeting the needs of the other. They find themselves trapped in limbo, unable to obtain the intimacy and affection they need from their spouses yet prohibited from seeking it elsewhere. They accumulate anger and resentment over their unmet needs. Quarreling ensues. Their injured feelings drive a wedge between them. They become isolated and emotionally disengaged and begin seeking emotional support and affection outside the marriage. This is, after all, what they are genetically programmed to do.

Now, the ex-lovers must make choices about engaging in infidelity. When a pair bond ends, the natural human inclination is to start looking for a new mate. Although marriage vows prohibit straying, people are genetically programmed to follow their instincts. Nonetheless, they feel guilty for showing interest in people other than their spouses, and they become angry when spouses have a "wandering eye." They accumulate resentment over broken promises made during the early stages of the pair bond, failing to recognize such promises are ephemeral. They equate infidelity with betrayal and rejection. Yet, if they do not stray, they regret their lost opportunities. They find themselves surrounded by unhappy, lonely humans who are in expired pairs or are unpaired, but they are obligated to keep all relationships outside their marriage non-romantic. They are permanently paired with someone they no longer love while restricted from reaching out to potential new lovers. This is often an insurmountable challenge.

If you fear loneliness, then do not marry.

— CHEKOV

Infidelity introduces more than just conflict into a marriage. It can sabotage the goal of monogamy by introducing questions of paternity. Uncertain paternity is the bane of extended parental investment. Fidelity was not important when humans were ignorant of paternity, relationships were brief, and new mates were just around the corner. However, when there is only one brood of offspring per lifetime, few men are willing to invest heavily in the future of children who are not theirs. It is a rare man who willingly pays for twenty years of food, lodging, clothing, auto insurance, and private school tuition for another man's children.

Maintaining an exhausted pair bond is difficult enough without all this bitterness. It is hard to provide support and affection when the desire to do so is gone. The additional burden of guilt and recrimination makes the task all but impossible. Couples come to feel they are in constant conflict with one another when, in fact, the real conflict is between their biological programming and their social obligations. Primitive instincts compel them to do things they know are not in the best interests of their children or their society. In advanced cultures, people stay together as couples for the sake of their children and their society. Staying together for the children is not a failure of the relationship. Rather, it indicates that the original pair bond has matured into a long-term post-romantic nuclear family.

Traditional Judeo-Christian marriage is an indefinite extension of the pair bond well into the post-romantic phase, and it places a great burden on a married couple. They must continue to behave as if they are pair-bonded when they are not. This is why so many couples feel their marriage is a sham. They are only pretending to be in love.

The extended relationship will be easier if couples understand that it is normal for lovers to lose interest when their pair bond matures. They must understand that they share many of the same sacrifices and discomforts and that these are simply the result of human nature. They should help each other overcome the loneliness, sadness, and regrets intrinsic to the extended rearing of children in contemporary society. They can do this by understanding each other's feelings and actively working to satisfy each other's needs, even after their natural inclination has diminished. They must transition to a new partnership based less on romance and more on friendship. It may help if each of them takes a few minutes each day to recall why they fell in love in the first place.

CHAPTER EIGHT

MAKING MONOGAMY WORK

It is not a lack of love, but a lack of friendship that makes unhappy marriages.

— FRIEDRICH NIETZSCHE

As a philosophy, monogamy has served humans well by providing extended parenting for children, but it is unnatural and uncomfortable. The belief that humans are naturally monogamous is detrimental for two reasons. First, when romance fades at the end of the pair bond, it leads to the shame, guilt, and resentment that destroy relationships. Second, it implies relationships hold themselves together spontaneously when, in fact, they do not. Cementing a post-romantic relationship requires a plan and an understanding of the differences between romantic and post-romantic bonds. The relationship becomes less of a love affair and more of a social partnership as romance fades.

Many marriages do last a lifetime. There are forces in the repertoire of human instincts and emotions that can maintain post-romantic relationships for half a century or more. Durable, long-

64

lasting partnerships are characterized by mutualism, respect, and reciprocity rather than passion.

All long-term partnerships have certain things in common. They are held together by basic human instincts that are not directly related to breeding. These same instincts are also present in romantic relationships, but they are completely overshadowed by the blinding passion of romance. Post-romantic couples and, for that matter, all non-romantic human relationships extending up to international politics are held together by altruism, reciprocity, empathy, shared kin, complementarity, and shared goals. They are constrained by inertia, fear of loss, loneliness, and fear of retribution. They are also affected by external social forces arising from religious beliefs, family expectations, and financial, legal, and moral obligations.

Reciprocal altruism is the inclination to help another person without expecting an immediate return, with the understanding that an eventual reciprocal service will occur. This is not unique to humans. It has been well documented in non-human primates. Reciprocal altruism is simple back-scratching. It is plain old-fashioned fairness. Successful couples help each other meet their separate goals. They support each other, provide for each other, and reciprocate their efforts toward the relationship. Couples take turns putting each other through college. They provide for each other's personal needs. They support each other through emotional crises and stroke each other's egos. They take turns doing the dishes. They do nice things for each other. They continue to invest in each other's welfare.

Reciprocal altruism is a philosophy about how members of a couple should treat each other. It underlies the recommendations in many relationship books about mutual respect, honesty, politeness, tolerance, and forgiveness. It is the Golden Rule and the basis of good friendship.

People will put up with all sorts of emotional insults and unfairness during the heat of passion, sacrificing a certain amount of their self-respect for the sake of the relationship. They are betting that what they gain from the relationship will eventually cover their losses. Once the opportunity to breed has passed and the initial passion is gone, the prospects for the future of a relationship are much less promising. Ex-lovers are much less forgiving of trespasses. Failure to adhere to the principles of reciprocal altruism in a post-romantic relationship drives a partner away.

Mature relationships survive best when people treat their partners as they would like to be treated. Reciprocity means each party to the relationship is fair to the other, meeting their responsibilities and accepting their share of the work of living together. They are truthful to one another in their words, body language, and actions. They are tolerant of what they see as faults in each other. They do not hold each other responsible for things beyond their control. They do not become angry at each other for being who they are or displaying their basic human emotions. They forgive each other's genuinely regretted misbehaviors and accept each other's sincere apologies.

<u>Kin altruism</u> is slightly different. It is the inclination to help one's relatives with no immediate reward to oneself, serving to increase family genes in the population. This is the basis of the social behaviors of ants, termites, and bees. The workers are all sisters. Only the queen lays eggs and produces young, while their older sisters, who forgo the opportunity to lay their eggs, care for the young. Kin altruism is the very heart of parenting. It is the reason that parents, aunts, uncles, and grandparents expend effort on child rearing.

This form of altruism is also important in selecting and caring for a mate. Humans generally choose mates who resemble the people from their childhood. It is a basic instinct. Men tend to choose women like their mothers in mannerisms, language, dress, and culture. Likewise, women tend to choose men who are like their fathers. People are more comfortable around people who resemble their relatives. People choose their mates from their society, culture, and community.

Kin altruism is the glue that binds social networks. A social network is the entire body of social contacts an individual possesses. It is the accumulated mass of a person's acquaintances and the inter-relationships of those acquaintances. Social networks are generally composed of persons from the same (or at least similar) cultures. When two people form a couple, they are not isolated individuals. They have social networks which will merge and need to be compatible.

People are instinctively more inclined to trust, help, empathize with, provide comfort and care for, ask directions from, and give directions to people who look familiar. They are more comfortable interacting with people who dress like them, speak their language, and have their facial features and skin color. They are more inclined to trust someone who looks like a family member, whether it involves dating, pair-bonding, marriage, business contracts, or apartment leases.

It should be readily apparent that prejudice is the absence of kin altruism, whether racial, ethnic, or religious. These two sentiments go hand in hand and are basic instincts in all human beings. People trust those who are familiar and mistrust those who are different. While contemporary cultures have made great progress in over-coming racial prejudice, it is still a large factor in reproductive rela-tionships. Couples who defy kin altruism and form mixed racial, ethnic, or religious pairs risk losing large portions of their social networks.

Empathy is the ability of one person to observe the actions of another, infer the emotions of that individual, and experience those emotions personally. People feel sad when seeing someone who is sad. They feel the suffering, humiliation, anger, and emotional pain of others. They also feel the others' joy, happiness, and relief. Empathy is what makes it possible for Hollywood and Disney to work their magic. When people observe actors or cartoon images on a screen, they can relate to the characters' emotions.

Empathetic individuals are aware of the feelings of others and consider them when interacting with a spouse. They try to avoid hurting each other's feelings. When people cry, others try to help because the crying makes them sad. When a woman cries because of her partner's actions, the partner may become sad and back-peddle on his position. When a man is upset over something his partner has said or done, she becomes sad and may alter her behavior.

Shared goals bond couples. This is different from reciprocal altruism. Altruism involves one person expending efforts toward the goals of another, while a shared goal means people are working on the same task together. Joint efforts toward common goals – whether it entails building a new house or just getting through the chores of another day – bind people together. The most important goal parents share is the rearing of their mutual offspring. This is the most frequently reported reason for preserving marriage in the absence of romance.

Couples share meals, hobbies, retirement goals, travel plans, houses, gardens, libraries, professional interests, woodworking projects, vacations, favorite foods, and favorite movies. They share good habits and bad habits. They share good times and disasters. They share friends and enemies. They share joys and chores. They share their experiences during the day and their emotions about the day. Parents share the raising of their children, preparing them to lead independent lives as adults. Finally, they hope to share the spoiling of their grandchildren. This is companionship, and it is the lifeblood of human relationships.

· · ·

<u>Complementarity</u> means people work together best when each can counter the shortcomings of the other. Humans tend to choose mates who have skills and talents that complement their own. That is, each member of the pair has abilities the other lacks. Complementarity strengthens a relationship. It may do so, in part, by providing ample opportunities for reciprocal altruism. Alternatively, each person may rely on the other for certain functions, and over time, they become so dependent on one another that they form a single functional unit. They are more financially stable and able to accomplish more together. Couples are under less stress when they have a high degree of complementarity.

This is reminiscent of the Chinese concept of Yin and Yang, the great duality of nature, in which two complementary parts form a whole. It reflects the Jewish concept of man and woman being two half-souls who form one complete soul when combined in marriage. It is the Christian ideal of two souls intertwined, two hearts that beat as one, bound together in a union sanctioned by God. It is a simple lesson taught by an old nursery rhyme.

> *Jack Spratt would eat no fat.*
> *His wife would eat no lean.*
> *And so betwixt the two of them,*
> *They picked the kettle clean.*

<u>Religion</u> is a relative newcomer to marriage. The institution of marriage preceded contemporary religion by many thousands of years. Marital relationships did not contain a spiritual component until two thousand years ago. Marriages were practical, social, and emotional arrangements. Religion assumed the dominant role in binding couples together by overseeing and sanctioning marriage. Judeo-Christian religions teach that falling in love and forming a pair bond identifies two people God created as soulmates or kindred spirits bound together for eternity. This creates a huge spiritual barrier that must be overcome before a Judeo-Christian person can

abandon a relationship. He or she must first invalidate the divine component of the union, usually by deciding that the original act of falling in love was unreal and the partner was misidentified as a soulmate.

Religion is a major factor in the selection of a mate. People define their sense of purpose and life goals based on their religious beliefs. Those are important shared concerns. Couples of the same religion share many other things: their basic values, social networks, and an afterlife for eternity. Religious congruity is a powerful positive stabilizing force in post-romantic relationships.

Religion binds couples through negative forces, too. Parties incur social costs when they break the bonds of matrimony. Religious couples may stay in relationships to avoid both the spiritual and the social consequences of defection. Abandoning a relationship may result in being shunned by one's religious community. This, in turn, results in the loss of a large part of one's social network, including relatives, business associates, and potential alternative mates. Some religions impose social restrictions or penalties on people who leave sanctioned marriages, which can be quite severe. Religious authorities can impose humiliation, banishment, death, and eternal damnation on those who leave a spouse or betray a sanctioned marriage through adultery or abandonment.

<u>Civil authorities</u>, likewise, place restrictions on the dissolution of the relationships they have sanctioned. The financial cost of divorce can be a significant barrier to couples, and many people end up separating without formal legal proceedings. In Western cultures, punitive measures are generally restricted to support payments and child custody arrangements, making it more difficult for the breadwinner to leave a marriage.

In Muslim cultures and some other strongly patriarchal Eastern and African societies, the laws are more punitive to women than men. A woman who leaves a marriage may be forced to pay large sums of money to her husband or his family. A woman who abandons her husband for another man may be imprisoned or executed.

<u>Inactivity Inertia</u> requires some explanation. The strongest forces binding relationships are internal, and the most pervasive of these is inactivity inertia. This concept is best illustrated by a small sea creature called a limpet, a little mollusk with a cone-shaped shell. Limpets live on rocks between the high and low tide lines on rocky seashores. They are grazers and generally roam only small distances from their home locations on the rocks, returning to their crevices each day. For many years, the question of whether limpets could move to a new home remained unanswered. Naturalists who study such things painted numbers on limpet shells, drew lines around them, and photographed them on their rocks every month. From this, they learned that limpets can move to a new home, but they generally do not. They mostly stay where they are.

The world is a dangerous place for limpets. If they get too close to the bottom of a rock, passing seabirds can stand on the sand at low tide and pry them off. If they get too low in the water, they are not exposed at low tide, and starfish will prey on them. If they get too high on the rock, they will not be covered at high tide and will dry out.

Limpets cannot see or hear. They cannot stand up and look into the distance. They cannot know what conditions will be like anywhere except where they are. They have no way of determining how safe another home might be, how far away it may be, or how hazardous the journey might be. Overall, if you are a limpet and are alive where you are, your best bet is just to stay there no matter how bad your local situation may be. For a limpet, the greatest safety lies in inactivity.

People are a lot like limpets. They tend to stay where they are, even when things might be better elsewhere. The reliability of their information about elsewhere is not as good as it is for their present location. The act of moving is dangerous and expensive. Unless the current situation is very bad or the promise of a new situation is very good, the move is not justified. People must overcome an inertial threshold before they activate change.

Inactivity inertia compels people to stay in bad relationships. This is why a woman stays with an ill-tempered, abusive, lazy husband or a man stays with a selfish, unloving, overspending wife. It is why nations keep bad governments and people stay in bad jobs. This is also why people who have been in their jobs for a long time are typically paid less than new hires in the same position. Business savvy employers know veteran employees are limpets who will not leave until the pay elsewhere is a great deal higher, while new employees require incentives to overcome their inertia and entice them to move. Likewise, abusive people have a sense of how much they can mistreat their spouses before they exceed the threshold for desertion.

Fear of retribution is a barrier that keeps couples together by preventing one or the other from leaving. Some people become abusive or punitive at any sign of disloyalty by a spouse. They mistreat spouses who show any inclination toward infidelity or desertion. This can take many forms: verbal abuse, relationship aggression, physical assault, and financial revenge. In extreme cases, one parent may mentally or physically abuse or even kill the children.

Fear of loss and loneliness can keep people together long after love is gone. They fear losing their home, property, and children. They fear losing their self-respect, social status, and social networks. They fear losing the investment they have made in their partner and the relationship.

Even a bad relationship provides some companionship and

escape from loneliness. Humans have a deeply rooted need for companionship. Regardless of their incompatibilities, two people have a lot in common when they are both lonely. No matter how emotionally impoverished a relationship may be, it is better than being alone. Most humans cannot thrive as solitary creatures.

To summarize, post-romantic relationships can persist in good health for decades, being maintained by a combination of forces, positive and negative, internal and external. The positive forces are reciprocal altruism, kin altruism, empathy, shared goals, and social networks. The negative forces are inactivity inertia, avoidance of loss, fear of retribution, and avoidance of loneliness. External pressures come from civil authorities and assert primarily negative forces in the form of penalties for the dissolution of relationships. Religion exerts positive forces by providing moral guidance and social networks, and it exerts negative pressures through punitive responses to adultery and desertion.

Every relationship is a unique combination of human interactions. Relationships are as varied as the human beings who form them. Generally, a good relationship is held together primarily by positive forces. Negative forces dominate a bad relationship. Unfortunately, where a given relationship falls is often unclear. Any relationship held together by consistently great sex and perfectly compatible social networks is good. Any relationship held together by mutual drug dependency, abuse, and fear of retribution is clearly bad.

However, most relationships contain a combination of positive and negative forces. They shift back and forth between good times and bad times, which is encouraging. It means that most troubled relationships can be improved easily. They can be nudged over to the good side, often with surprisingly little effort. It just takes a basic understanding of the principles involved and a willingness to apply them.

A great wealth of advice can be found in the "Relationships" section of any bookstore, but it is difficult to implement in the setting of shame, guilt, and resentment that often dominates a failing relationship. If people understood why a pair bond ends, why they fall out of love, and why their ego boundaries return, then they would be in a much better position to adopt sound relationship guidance.

Remember, incredible as it may seem, this is what humans do under natural conditions. Humans are instinctively programmed to separate after a few years and go on to find new mates. It should not be surprising so many marriages fail to last a lifetime. Rather, it should be surprising so many last as long as they do. It is sad that so many couples are led to believe they have personally failed when they stop loving each other. They become entangled in emotional turmoil and drama. Their shame, guilt, and resentment prevent them from working together constructively. They fail to gain insight into the causes of their animosity, leaving them doomed to repeat their mistakes in the next relationship.

A great deal of human suffering can be avoided if young people are taught that they are not truly designed to stay together as life-long couples. There are good reasons for them to stay together, but it is not natural. We humans are genetically programmed to leave behind a trail of ex-lovers and to remain on good terms with them. Indigenous people continued living in the same village or forest, sharing the raising of children and respecting and caring for each other long after their pair bonds ended. Remember, the whole point of the process was and still is to raise healthy children who can populate the next generation. Any sexual strategy that results in a new crop of well-adjusted adults is a biological success, whether it lasts for four years or forty.

My good friend Katlyn is a wonderful example. She divorced a few years ago and lamented how ashamed and embarrassed she felt over the failure of her marriage. She and her husband were married for twenty-three years and raised two sons who completed undergraduate college degrees. I counseled her that she was unfairly crit-ical of herself and her husband. The two of them have raised their children well. They have completed an entirely successful marriage. They should congratulate each other over a bottle of champagne and celebrate their achievement, then feel free to separate and find love again with whomever they wish. If they can discard their shame, guilt, and resentment, they may even find love again with each other.

Kissing don't last, cookery do.

— GEORGE MEREDITH

CHAPTER NINE
MARRIAGE: SOCIAL BONDING

And a man shall leave his mother
And a woman leave her home
And they shall travel on to where
The two shall be as one.

— THE WEDDING SONG, BY NOEL "PAUL"
STOOKEY

THREE WESTERN DEFINITIONS OF MARRIAGE:

New Webster's Dictionary, 1993: "The institution under which a man and a woman become legally united on a permanent basis."

...short and simple

Oxford English Dictionary, 1971: "The condition of being husband and wife. The relationship between married persons. Spousehood. Wedlock."

... Followed by a 3600-word discourse on etymology and variations.

Wikipedia.com, 2009: "Marriage is a social, spiritual, and/or legal union of individuals. ... an institution in which interpersonal relationships (usually intimate and sexual) are acknowledged by the state, by religious authority, or by both."

... Note the absence of gender and number.

Marriage is a ubiquitous behavior among humans. Some form of marriage is recognized in every culture, no matter how primitive or advanced. It ranges from informal, personal, private declarations to internationally witnessed and sanctioned events that bind the fortunes of great nations and huge populations. It may last only as long as the couple wishes or until the end of not only their lives but the lives of their descendants. It can be a simple agreement between two lovers or an arrangement involving their families, communities, local political entities, religious authorities, sovereign states, and international immigration boards. It may be sexually exclusive, completely "open," or anything in between. The two parties may be intimate lovers or strangers. Some marriages do not include any arrangement for sexual activity at all, and some married couples never meet.

VARIOUS PERSPECTIVES ON MARRIAGE

The highest happiness on Earth is marriage

— WILLIAM LYON PHELPS

What a happy and holy fashion it is that those who love one another should rest on the same pillow.

— NATHANIAL HAWTHORNE

I've been married eleven years and I've had three children. I guess that means I breed well in captivity.

— ROSEANNE BARR

Any intelligent woman who reads the marriage contract, and then goes into it, deserves all the consequences.

— ISADORA DUNCAN

Marriage Ceremony: An incredible physical sham of watching God and the law being dragged into the affairs of your family.

— O.C. OGILVIE

People tend to have a narrow view of marriage based on their own culture. For the industrialized Western world, this generally means marriage is between two people – a man and a woman – and it occurs when they fall in love and decide to raise a family. However, in the overall theater of humanity, most marriages are between two people who are not in love, and most people who fall in love do not marry. Furthermore, most children are not raised within the shelter of marriage. Many marriages are not confined to one man and one woman, and many do not include both sexes in the union.

The 2006 National Vital Statistics Report revealed that thirty-eight percent of children are born out of wedlock in the United States, where the law endorses typical Judeo-Christian marriage traditions. This is up from thirty-two percent in 1996 and twenty-three percent in 1986. Worldwide, the out-of-wedlock birth rate is about twenty-five percent, based on figures compiled in the late 1990s. When these figures are added to the divorce rates for couples with children, more than half of the world's children have single parents or stepparents.

The increase in single motherhood in Western culture is primarily among women in their twenties and thirties who have chosen to be single mothers, rather than among teenagers, who presumably just do not know any better. More women choose single motherhood partly because new liberal views on sexuality make it difficult to secure a traditional husband. The great majority of the births to unwed mothers are the product of loving relationships that did not advance to marriage. Humans fall in love many more times than they marry. Marriage is no longer required or expected for the parents of a child. Marriage is also no longer an expected outcome of falling in love. The great majority of human pair bonds end before marriage occurs. Generally, people need more reason to marry than just falling in love or having a child.

My young colleague, Dan, was head over heels in love with one of his classmates, Alicia, in their senior year in college. They lived together all through graduate school but did not marry. As they approached graduation during their fourth year, they began to quarrel about their final professional destinations. This issue divided them, and they went their separate ways.

The love affair between Dan and Alicia illustrates the pair-bonding duration. Their pair bond lasted four years and ended over an issue that would have been insignificant in the first year of their relationship. Their ego boundaries had returned, and these two people no longer wanted each other enough to sacrifice their professional aspirations for the sake of their relationship.

This case illustrates the importance of extrinsic factors in marriage. These two people were very much in love. They were intensely pair-bonded, but they were not at the right time and place in their lives for marriage. They put it off for too long, and the opportunity expired.

Of course, marriage does not need to be based on love at all. Arranged marriages between children or adults who may have never met are common in many modern cultures. Couples are marrying somewhere in the world today who are being introduced for the first time at the wedding ceremony.

In Western culture, marriage is historically defined as a male-female dyad, but that is a local tradition only. Restricting the definition of marriage to only one arrangement has no anthropological basis. It is purely a matter of cultural preferences, or a local option, usually imposed by tradition and supported by religion. See *Sex Rules* by Brodman (2017) for a delightful tour through the diverse sex and marriage customs of existing indigenous cultures. Here are a few variations on the concept of marriage.

1. One man and one woman – Sexually exclusive: This is the standard Judeo-Christian marriage. It first appeared in the fourth century in Christian Europe (Lewis, 2009) and became the norm by the tenth century. It is now common in all modern cultures, where it is referred to as monogamy or the nuclear family.

2. One man and one woman – Not sexually exclusive: Primitive hunter-gatherers and prehistoric people formed pair bonds but accepted infidelity (Ryan, 2010). This type of marriage persists in many aboriginal cultures (Fielding, 1942). In modern society, it is known as an "open relationship" or "open dyad." In the extreme, it is polyamory (see below).

3. One man and several women – Polygynous marriage was common throughout history and is still practiced in the Muslim religion and many indigenous cultures (Lee, 1993; Tonkinson, 1991; van den Berghe, 1990).

4. One woman and several men – This is polyandrous marriage and is traditional in Nepal and Northern India, usually involving fraternal polyandry when several brothers share one wife (Fielding, 1942; van den Berghe, 1990).

5. One woman and several women – Among the American Plains Indians, some women became warriors and took one or more wives (Ewers, 1961, pp 185-190).

6. Several men and several women – In some aboriginal cultures, groups of adults are married, such as a group of brothers in one family or a group of sisters in another, known as group marriage (van der Berghe, 1990). In the modern world, this type of relationship is known as polyamory. Many resources for polyamory can be found on the Internet (polyamory.org; polyamory.com; polyamorysociety.org).

7. Two women (or two men) – Same-sex marriage is currently controversial and undergoing radical change worldwide. Historically, same-sex marriage has been documented for eons. See Hinsch (1990) and Boswell (1995) for examples in ancient Rome and China.

8. One woman and one tree – This is a Hindu custom allowing a woman to escape a common type of astrological curse (Sundarum, 2007).

9. One man and one tree – This is also a Hindu marriage tradition related to the belief that an older brother should marry first. When a young man wants to marry, but his older brother is unmarried, the older brother may be married to a tree. This clears the way for the younger brother to marry a woman (Fielding, 1942).

10. One man and one deity – Ancient Sumerian kings married female deities, as did some Celtic kings.

11. One woman and one deity – Catholic nuns in some orders, such as the Franciscan Sisters, are married to Christ (www.torsisters.com/faq.htm).

12. Marriage without sex – This is known as a spiritual marriage, or a Josephite marriage, in the Catholic church.

13. Arranged marriage – Common throughout the world in both modern and ancient cultures. (Tonkinson, 1991; van

den Berghe, 1990). Even today, the great majority of Hindu marriages in India are arranged. (Hawley, 2007, pp. 63-75.)

14. Child marriage – Historically, children have been the subject of betrothals in every conceivable combination. Children are betrothed not only to other children but also to adults (Tonkinson, 1991; van den Berghe, 1990). In some extreme cultures, unborn females were wed to adult males (Fielding, 1942; Janssen, 2002). Child marriages have now been illegalized in much of the Western world and Asia, but still occur in India and Australasia, and, surprisingly, in the United States (Wikipedia: Child Marriage in the United States.)

Love is recognized in nearly every culture, but it is not always relevant to marriage. In Western societies, most people who marry are in love, but that was not true for several thousand years of human history. Even today, love is rarely enough for two people to wed. As with Dan and Alicia, two people who marry must be at the right time and place in both of their lives. They must clear their playing fields of other potential or former mates. They need the financial ability and legal freedom to marry. Their social networks should be compatible and encourage marriage. Generally, one or more incentives from the following list will contribute to their decision.

Related to child-rearing

- Creating an extended pair bond to raise children
- Formation of a legal family unit
- Securing a sexual partner for procreation
- Social stability for children born out of wedlock to a couple

- Procurement of a mother/father for children of a single man/woman
- Procurement of a provider for children of a single parent
- Meeting requirements for adoption of children
- Meeting moral/religious/ethical obligations for an unintended pregnancy

Relating to sex

- Securing a sexual partner, not for procreation
- Legitimizing sexual relations with an existing partner

Related to intra-sex competition

- Finalizing the outcome of competition for a mate
- Securing a trophy spouse
- Establishing a legal barrier against adversaries for a sexual partner

Related to property holdings

- Obtaining pension benefits
- Securing an inheritance or other property
- Securing control of property or business that is not owned
- Merging personal property to improve lifestyle

Related to legal benefits

- Improving military benefits
- Avoiding military deployment
- Obtaining medical insurance coverage
- Obtaining citizenship
- Securing residency other than citizenship

- Securing or obtaining social security benefits
- Reducing taxes
- Meeting qualifications for a mortgage or other housing

Related to the public persona

- Publicly declaring love
- Publicly declaring heterosexuality
- Publicly declaring homosexuality
- Performing a publicity stunt
- Publicly declaring "normalcy"

Related to social standing

- Merging political interests of different families
- Social climbing
- Fulfilling religious obligations

Related to personal safety

- Shotgun weddings
- Procuring protection for a woman and her children

Related to personal loss

- Filling the void left by the loss of a spouse
- Filling the void left by the loss of a parent

Related to scripting

- Meeting perceived parental or community expectations
- Following the example set by older siblings

REPRODUCTIVE BONDING PRECEDES HUMANS

The social and sexual relationships of gorillas, baboons, chimpanzees, and bonobos demonstrate some surprisingly human attributes.

<u>Gorillas</u> live in groups that include one dominant male, two to seven females, and their juvenile offspring. The male bonds with females for life. The females and young stay close to the dominant male and rely on him for protection from predators and free-roaming male gorillas. The dominant males are highly protective of their females and the juveniles they have sired, but male gorillas may sometimes kill juveniles who are not their offspring.

Adolescent males and females leave the troop to find mates. A female may join another group, or a male and two or more females may form a new group. Females have a twenty-eight-day menstrual cycle. They initiate sexual activity when they are in estrus. Males do not initiate sex.

<u>Baboons</u> live in large troops of up to several hundred individuals. A group will typically consist of several dominant males, each of which will have a harem of up to five females. These males will jealously guard their females and mistreat them if they stray too far. They will bite and strike females who wander too close to another male.

However, some individuals engage in an alternate mating strategy. A single male and female may form a special bond and stay on the periphery of the troop. This male helps his female find food and will share his food with an infant in her care. He defends her and the infant from other males and predators. When she is in estrus, she mates exclusively with him. In the animal behavior literature, the baboons who form these pairs are called "special friends," but their relationship is clearly a primitive romance.

. . .

<u>Chimpanzees</u> live in troops of 50 to 150 and are highly promiscuous. The female has a thirty-six-day menstrual cycle. Her rump becomes red and swollen during estrus, advertising her availability to adult males. At this time, the males may line up to copulate with her. Interestingly, males and females who are closely related will not copulate. However, the family structure is matrilineal. That is, the chimps know who their mothers are, but in such a promiscuous society, they cannot know their fathers. A female chimp will not mate with her son or brother, but she will very likely copulate with her father, just by chance, because she does not know his identity and is likely to copulate with every male in the group at some time.

Chimps are highly territorial, and a single animal or small group who wanders into a neighboring territory will almost certainly be killed. However, a female in estrus uses her swollen rump like a passport to migrate freely to another group or territory. Her willingness to submit to sex redirects the aggressive energy of males.

Like baboons, chimps sometimes have special friends. Occasionally, a single male and female will leave the troop for a time. They will go off in the jungle by themselves for up to three months, foraging and grooming. This male will have a monopoly on the female in estrus. Unlike the special friendship of the baboon pair, the developing romance of the chimps ends once the female becomes pregnant.

<u>Bonobos</u>, also called pygmy chimpanzees, are the most promiscuous of the primates. These creatures have sex constantly. They have sex as a greeting or when they share food. They use sex to establish rank, soothe hurt feelings, mend relationships, and resolve conflicts. Both males and females masturbate frequently. There is no bonding between individual adults for reproduction.

Sex among bonobos appears completely unrestricted. It is as

common among juveniles as it is among adults. Both males and females initiate sex. Homosexual copulation is as common as heterosexual couplings. Sex is performed in the missionary position as often as any other position, and the couples kiss with their lips and tongue. Sex is not restricted to estrus but is practiced throughout the female menstrual cycle, although the female will initiate sex more frequently when she is in estrus than at other times. Female bonobos have been documented to engage in sex with males in exchange for food.

Many elements of human mating behavior can be observed among these four primate groups. Baboons and chimps form temporary pair bonds based on the provision of resources and protection for the female in return for exclusive sexual access for the male. Gorillas form life-long bonds in a polygynous arrangement. The male gorillas and baboons protect and care for the offspring of the females in their company. Female chimps use sex to redirect male aggression and enter new social groups. Both bonobos and chimps use their sexuality for various social purposes other than reproduction. Both males and females use sex to establish political alliances and determine rank in their groups. Bonobos engage in sex purely for pleasure or as a form of play. These four primates display a wide range of behaviors seen in human relationships, including romance, cooperation, pairing, protection, faithfulness, devotion, compromise, sex play, and homosexuality. They also include promiscuity, polyandry, polygyny, jealousy, oppression, spouse abuse, incest, and abandonment.

PREHISTORIC HUMAN MARRIAGE

Even the oldest, most primitive human cultures have well-established marriage customs that specify sexual obligations. However, it is important to note that those sexual obligations are completely unrelated to reproduction. They are for social bonding. Primitive humans did not engage in sex to have children. They did not know the connection. At the dawn of human history, pregnancy was thought to come from spirits or to occur spontaneously.

Humans did not acquire knowledge of the relationship between sex and conception until they domesticated animals. Before that time, sex had a purely social function. It helped determine who was friendly to whom, who shared food and resources, who stood where in the pecking order of the group, and who would take sides with whom during a group conflict. Pregnancy, on the other hand, just happened by itself.

HUNTER-GATHERER SOCIETIES

The Mardu Aborigines in the Western Desert of Australia know how babies occur. A woman becomes pregnant when a spirit child enters her body through her mouth, nose, or vagina. Spirit children are present all around the Mardu in the plants and animals and in the sacred places. The Mardu know when a woman receives a spirit child because she vomits some food she has eaten. If she eats some kangaroo and vomits, then a spirit child has come from the kangaroo and entered her body. The spirit will grow into a baby, exit her body, and become a person. It will live a life as a human and will then return to the spirit world when the human dies.

Like most primitive hunter-gatherers, the Mardu do not recognize any cause-and-effect relationship between sex and pregnancy. They have no concept of paternity and no awareness of any part played by a male in the pregnancy. In fact, they do not understand the role played by the mother. They believe the spirit child feeds itself until birth and is sometimes accidentally born to the wrong mother.

Mardu Aboriginal marriages are arranged between young adult males and prepubescent girls. Mardu children are well aware of sex and often play sexual games that may even include coitus. A married girl may continue to play these games with other children but will not begin sexual activity with her husband until she begins to have menses. Sexual relations between a husband and wife are a social obligation among the Mardu, but they are not exclusive, and they are not related to child-rearing. The Mardu marriages are "open" marriages in the sense that both partners are free to engage in sex with any other person they choose. No one objects unless the infidelity leads to elopement. Marriages in the Mardu community are arranged years in advance and are the basis of the community's social structure. An elopement threatens that structure. Paradoxically, the Mardu have a very liberal view of infidelity, but they view falling in love as a threat to domestic tranquility.

Among the Yanomami, a group of hunter-gatherers in South America, marriages are arranged in a cross-cousin pattern within the village or arranged with a partner in an adjacent village for political gain and reduced risk of warfare. Pubescent girls at menarche are wed to young men in their twenties.

The Yanomami believe men play an important role in pregnancy. This culture teaches that the unborn baby is nourished by semen. The healthiest babies are born to mothers who have the most sexual encounters during pregnancy. Many men in the community play a role in a woman's pregnancy by providing food to the mother and feeding her baby through copulation. Yanomami culture does not recognize the actual role of semen in conception. All the men who have sex with a woman during pregnancy are equally responsible for the baby's well-being. Yanomami marry, and the marriage partners have sexual obligations, but they are free to engage in sex with others.

The !Kung San, a.k.a. the Kalahari bushmen, are an ancient people who still live in groups of up to a hundred in the Kalahari Desert in Central Africa. They live a nomadic hunter-gatherer lifestyle, with each group confined to a territory. They have well-established marriage customs, including both arranged marriages and pair-bonding. The group holds a ceremony to witness a marriage. The first marriage is arranged between an older woman and a young man and is usually short-lived. Subsequent marriages are pair bonds. They last a few years each. Marriages are dissolved privately and informally.

As in other hunter-gatherer cultures, marriage among the !Kung San is not sexually exclusive. Men and women have sexual obligations to their marriage partners, but they are free to have sex with whomever they choose. Infidelity is generally done discreetly. Even where promiscuity is the norm, too much blatant infidelity can precipitate a conflict with a spouse and/or a rival. In such cultures, jealousy is frowned upon, and the group may chastise a male who makes too much fuss over his wife's infidelity. Even so, fighting over women is the most common cause of homicide among the !Kung San.

!Kung San believe the wife must give sex to the husband and care for the children. The husband helps care for his wife's children to the extent he wishes, although he is not obligated to do that. His obligation is to provide meat and other resources to the woman. The wife also provides food in the form of plant products she gathers. The !Kung San frankly state that if a wife wants to be rid of her husband, she only needs to refuse him sex and he will leave. If a husband wants to be free of his wife, he needs only stop providing for her, and she will abandon him.

As in most hunter-gatherer cultures, !Kung San children nurse from their mothers' breasts for two to three years. Subsequently, the village raises them. A typical !Kung San adult has four or five marriages throughout a lifetime, with one or two children per marriage. Only two of these children, on average, will survive to reproductive age.

Hunter-gatherer cultures are promiscuous and have no concept of paternity, as in the Mardu, or a very inaccurate concept, as in the Yanomami. In these cultures, as in the great apes, incest taboos exist but are limited by the lack of a basic understanding of fatherhood. The taboos restrict women from engaging in sex with their brothers and sons but not with their fathers because they do not know the identity of their fathers. Likewise, men do not engage in sex with their sisters or mothers, but they may engage in sex with their biological daughters simply because they cannot know which young women in the community are their daughters.

The danger of accidental liaisons between father and daughter persists today among promiscuous humans. It was a sub-plot of the movie *Rumor Has It,* starring Jennifer Aniston and Kevin Costner. Released in 2005, the film tells of a brief affair between Sarah and an older man named Beau, which creates havoc when Sarah discovers her mother had an affair with Beau about the time she was conceived. She is horrified that she might have accidentally had sex with her biological father. Of course, the matter is resolved before the end of the film, but the presence of this theme in a popular film shows public awareness of this particular social hazard in promiscuous populations.

HOE-BASED AGRICULTURE SOCIETIES

About ten thousand years ago, humans began practicing crude agriculture. As humans transitioned from hunter-gatherers to hoe-based agricultural societies, they settled into villages. Women had homes and tended small gardens. They were bound to the land. A woman and her children would till and plant a small plot of land using only hand tools, such as hoes and digging sticks.

The women cultivated vegetables, while men hunted and provided meat for the women and their children. The meat constituted less than half of the calories but provided most of the dietary protein essential for children's health. Men also provided other resources and services to earn their keep. Men could physically protect women and their children from wild animals or human interlopers. They could handle heavy objects and build shelters.

The women competed for the services of men. A woman with many children had many helping hands to work the garden. Her value was based on her fecundity or her ability to bear children. A younger woman without children was a greater risk. She might be barren and evil. Under primitive conditions, when a man considered a woman as a mate, pre-existing children were a plus.

This was and still is the matrilineal, matrilocal family. It persists today in many areas of the world. Marriages were informal arrangements in which a man took up residence with a woman for a while, helping her raise her children while having relatively exclusive sexual access to her. The pair bond continued until he got tired of the domestic life or until she got tired of him and ran him off. He would then go off to stay by himself or take up with another woman. In time, another man would take his place.

None of these men knew which children were his. The children would refer to any one of the men in their lives as their father. A woman kept a man close to her by giving him companionship and affection, and he earned his keep by giving her companionship, resources, and protection. She would likely become pregnant by him in the process, and both their genes would be propagated.

Note that up to this point in human history, females owned all wealth, including land, housing, and children. Women were free to have sex with whomever they chose. Men were transient in their lives. This was the reproductive lifestyle to which humans were adapted, whether by evolution or design. Until about seven thousand years ago, this is how humans naturally paired and reproduced.

Let me reiterate this point because it is so important. Prehistoric men did not own families. Women were in charge of property, families, and their sexuality. They had freedom to engage in sex with whomever they wished and used that sex to get what they wanted from the men around them.

COWS, PLOWS, AND THE DEMISE OF WOMEN'S RIGHTS

About seven thousand years ago, humans developed plows and large-scale agriculture. According to Helen Fisher in *The Anatomy of Love*, this was a disaster for women. Plowing was done with oxen and horses and required the strength of men. Once land was tilled, the land itself became valuable. A piece of arable land had to be defended from marauders, and defense of the land required men.

When humans domesticated animals, they became aware of the relationship between sex and offspring. They learned to recognize paternal lineages in their stock and their own families. They began to guard their wives.

Large-scale agriculture and animal husbandry concentrated the food production industry into a small population. It freed people from subsistence hunting and gardening and allowed the emergence of skilled artisans. The products of these craftsmen were traded over long distances, and commerce was born.

As landowners, artisans, and merchants accumulated wealth, they started to obsess about inheritance. Land and wealth had to be defended by men, had to belong to men, and had to be inherited by their sons.

The role of women changed drastically. Their value was no longer determined by their ability to produce many children but by their ability to produce children of known paternity. A woman's value was no longer determined by fecundity, but rather by fidelity. She was no longer expected to be prolific, but rather to be chaste. Women lost the freedom to choose their mates or change sexual partners. They lost all opportunities to engage in extramarital sex or premarital sex. They were mandated to practice abstinence until marriage. All of their mating choices were made by men. They were forced to be faithful to the men who provided their livelihoods and severely punished for any deviation from the rules laid down by men.

Women became pieces of the estate. They were the property of their male kin. A woman was the soil in which a man planted his seed. She was subservient not only to her husband/owner but also to her father, brothers, and sons. Her male kin chose her sexual partner. Marriages were contracts between families. The marriage certificate was a property deed, not much different than a bill of sale for a horse.

The oldest known written laws describing marriage are in the Hammurabi Code, written in Babylon 3750 years ago. These describe marriage as a commercial transaction for the sale and ownership of women. Husbands bought and sold wives. These women were their property. Men could imprison their wives or put them in chains. A husband could purchase a new wife and downgrade the status of his current wife to a household slave.

The past century has seen major changes in the Western world, with women no longer being the personal possessions of men. However, residual traditions still reflect a time when women were property. The old beliefs and values persist as subtle intrusions in our culture. Tradition still dictates a suitor request the permission of the bride's father for his daughter's hand in marriage. The father escorts the bride to the altar, reminiscent of a time when she would not have gone willingly. The father (the current owner) gives away his daughter (his property) to the groom (the new owner). The bride is expected to be a virgin, dressed in white, while the groom is not. The bride is carried across the threshold, reminiscent of a time when she would not have gone into the man's home willingly.

A wife is expected to adhere to absolute fidelity, while the husband is not. In many places today, an unfaithful wife is still severely punished, while an adulterous husband is begrudgingly tolerated. Adultery by the wife is universally considered grounds for divorce, while adultery by the husband is not. Even in Western cultures today, a wife is financially penalized for adultery. In most of the United States, the laws regarding spousal support are punitive towards a married woman who exercises sexual freedom. In divorce proceedings, a woman who was supported by her husband during the marriage is entitled to continued support after the divorce in the form of alimony. However, if a woman commits adultery during the marriage, she does not get alimony.

• • •

Religion was a latecomer in the marriage business. About 2000 years ago, the Jewish faith decreed that man and woman were only partial souls who merged through marriage to form a complete soul. About 1300 years ago, Muhammad revealed Allah's rules regarding how many wives a man could have, how he should treat them, and how they should treat him. About 1100 years ago, the Catholic Church sanctified marriage as a "Holy Union" and introduced the concept of "till death do we part." Marriage became a spiritual union sanctioned by a deity and persisting throughout life and into eternity.

About 1000 years ago in Europe, landlords began to exercise control over peasant marriages as a land-management tool. Formal registration and licensing of marriages by local government began about 400 years ago in Europe. Authorities had good reasons to take an interest in marriage. As humans accumulated personal wealth, marriage became a legal device for transferring property through inheritance. Transfers of property and money are opportunities for taxation, which is always an incentive for civil authorities to exert control. Moreover, marriage became a political tool to create alliances when land and political power were inherited, so authorities encouraged people to stay with their marriage partners to maintain the political structure.

Today, the government's interest in marriage focuses on protecting the rights of any children born in the marriage, but this is a very modern innovation. Until a century ago, the government did not show any interest in the welfare of children. They were simply the property of their father, to be treated as he wished and disposed of as he pleased. This changed in 1924 when the League of Nations proclaimed the rights of children to receive food, shelter, medical care, and protection from abuse and exploitation. The United Nations expanded on this in 1959 with their Declarations of the Right of the Child.

THE GENDER OF GOD

Before the domestication of animals, all gods were female. Women were the creators of humanity and the universe. All life sprang forth from the womb of a woman. All creation myths credited a female, an Earth Mother, under many different names. Goddesses controlled the fates of humans and their world. Venus figurines are small stone or ivory effigies of the Mother Goddess. Hundreds have been found, spanning from 45,000 years ago to 11,000 years ago. No male figurines have ever been found from that time period.

Gradually, beginning about 7000 years ago, the gender of the gods began to change. As people learned about the relationship between sex and pregnancy, the all-female roster of gods began to acquire male consorts. These consorts were not gods themselves but were in service to their goddesses. Some were the sons of the Goddesses. Many were replaced annually. They were transients in the great halls of the female deities. See *When God was a Woman*, by Merlin Stone, for a complete discussion.

Over time, as men came to dominate family life, deities changed. Male consorts acquired more power and influence. They became kings appointed by the female goddesses. Many ancient mythologies share a common theme of the male consort killing the female god to seize power. The female deities shifted away from the role of givers of life and became associated with evil, darkness, and snakes. The myths report how male deities achieved domination by overcoming the seductions and deceits of women.

The invention of large-scale agriculture enabled another revolution, the provision and feeding of armies. Previously, when agriculture was hand-to-mouth, there were no professional soldiers. Warfare was small-scale between rival villages, as it still is today among the Yanomamo or the Mardu. Cultural expansion occurred through the gradual migration of people or the adoption of ideas by neighbors. The emergence of large-scale agriculture allowed the formation of political units that could support organized military forces. These were, of course, dominated by men. Cultures began to change much more rapidly through military campaigns rather than simple migration. These military invaders brought their male gods with them.

This is well documented in the Middle East and Anatolia, areas overrun by intruders from the Russian steppes with their domesticated horses and newly invented chariots and swords. These invaders from the north brought patriarchal cultures and gods, extinguishing matriarchal cultures in their path. They beget the first male monotheist religion, Zoroastrianism. It advanced with them across the Anatolian peninsula and into the Middle East. The Israelites adopted the idea when they were exiled to Babylon, and they carried it back to their eventual homeland, where it became the backbone of the three Abrahamic religions. These three religions, Judaism, Islam, and Christianity, share the same male deity and patriarchal culture inherited from Zoroastrianism.

The final blow to female deities in the Middle East came when the Israelites conquered the Hittites and Canaanites, who still worshiped female gods. With a male deity and an all-male cast of prophets and kings, the Israelites wiped out the last of the goddess worshipers about 3000 years ago. Many scholars interpret the tale of Adam's seduction by Eve in the Garden of Eden and the female culpability for all the woes of humanity as propaganda warning the Israelite men of the dangerous priestesses lurking in the Hittite and Canaanite houses of worship. It is also a clear statement of the subservient role the Israelite male god intended for women.

Women lost their human rights and the control of families, and female gods lost the power to control human populations. Families and religions became patriarchal. Women lost all influence over worship, government, and their reproductive choices. Their rights became the whims of male gods and the men who interpreted those whims. Yet, even today, we still recognize the role of a female as the divine nurturer and creator under the name of Mother Nature.

ENFORCEMENT OF FIDELITY

As wealth and political power accumulated, the motivation to enforce marriage vows increased. The primary objective of this enforcement effort was control of paternity. The husband must always be the father of any children of the marriage.

The maternity of a child is never in question. Everyone in the community knows whose birth canal delivered a baby. Paternity is not so certain. Restrictions had to be placed on women to ensure that any child born to a woman was fathered by her husband. A double standard in sexual freedoms arose from the cultural transition that occurred 7000 years ago. When inheritances were involved, paternity of heirs needed to be controlled at all costs, but the costs were mostly levied upon women.

Marriage meant the eventual transfer of property to the children of the wife. The wealth a man and his ancestors had accumulated must not go to another man's offspring. It became essential that husbands prevent their wives from becoming pregnant by other men. The husbands must not be cuckolded. From the male point of view, a married woman who bore a male child of a man other than her husband was committing an act of great thievery. She was stealing all the accumulated wealth of her husband and all his ancestors, and she deserved severe punishment.

The belief that men should control who impregnates the women in their community is biologically flawed. It stands in stark defiance of the natural order. It is an attempt to override sexual selection. Under natural conditions, females are supposed to decide which males reproduce, and males are supposed to decide which females reproduce. The modern rules of marriage, which apply fidelity only to females, attempt to usurp the natural privileges of females. It is a violation of some very basic rules of biology. Mother Nature would not approve.

The determination of men to pursue this objective has led to some very peculiar – and sometimes gruesome – consequences in the historical record. Some cultures have encouraged infanticide of firstborn children. Both men and women have been imprisoned or mutilated. Cruel and horrible punishments have been meted out, all in the name of preserving morality while ensuring the legitimacy of heirs. Countless women have been executed for the crime of adultery, and the practice continues today in some cultures, most recently under fundamentalist Muslim regimes. European noblemen put their women in iron chastity belts. Some extant Islamic cultures still keep women imprisoned and force them to wear dehumanizing outer garments. Female genital mutilation persists in much of Africa and the Middle East. This renders the female incapable of enjoying sex and often results in painful sex. In some cultures, the wife's labia majora are sewn together. The stitches are released only long enough for the husband to have sex with her. Then, the opening is re-sewn.

The use of brutal methods to control sexuality in females has not been limited to Muslims. Clitorectomy, the surgical removal of the clitoris, was an accepted treatment for many female childhood disorders, including excessive sexuality in young girls in Victorian England and the United States, well into the twentieth century. The last well-respected medical textbook to recommend clitorectomy to treat female childhood masturbation was published in 1936. Less than a century ago, genital mutilation of females was still prescribed in England and the United States.

TERMINATION OF MARRIAGES

Wherever there has been marriage, there has also been divorce. In most primitive cultures, either party to marriage could end a union, and the process was often informal. Until the last century, most post-Neolithic cultures only allowed men to initiate divorce. Men have universally been allowed to divorce women who engaged in adultery. However, adultery has rarely been accepted as a cause for women to divorce their husbands.

Conversely, non-support has been widely accepted as a cause for women to divorce their husbands but has rarely been a cause for husbands to divorce their wives. Generally, when marriage included an informal arrangement, divorce was casual. Late in the game, as religious and civil authorities became involved in marriage, they also exerted control over divorce.

In cultures where men owned everything, women left the marriage with nothing. They might have returned to their parents or lived on the streets. Some cultures allowed them to be downgraded to the status of a household slave. In some cultures, a woman's jewelry and dowry were her property. In others, she might have retained her inheritance from her parents. In matrilineal, matrilocal societies, the children stayed with their mothers. In patrilineal cultures, children were the property of the father. They did not remain with the mother unless they were thought to be the product of an adulterous union. This remained the case well into the nineteenth century.

THE CURRENT STATE OF MARRIAGE AND GENDER ROLES

The past century has witnessed tremendous upheaval in marriage traditions and reproductive behavior in the Western world. Young people who read this paragraph today cannot possibly fathom the changes that have occurred in the past century. In the 1920s, the pioneering work of Margaret Sanger initiated a revolution in human reproduction and the course of human history. Prior to her efforts, birth control devices were illegal in many states, and literature on birth control was classified as obscene and unlawful. Her efforts culminated in the legalization of birth control in 1965. Until a mere century ago, women in the United States were not legally allowed to avoid pregnancy and child-rearing.

By contrast, women in the Western world today choose their sexual partners, make their own reproductive decisions, and exercise complete control over whether, when, and by whom they become pregnant. Women can no longer be forced into marriage in European and Western cultures. They choose their own spouses and lovers. They need the consent of their parents only if they are juveniles.

Nonetheless, arranged marriage customs persist in large areas of the world. Some nations and religions still allow the reproductive choices of both males and females to be made by relatives without any regard for the feelings of the soon-to-be sexual partners. The Hindu culture has eight marriage types, and seven of them are arranged by relatives. A third party arranges more than seventy-five percent of marriages in present-day India. It is worth noting that most Hindus outside of India have abandoned this practice.

Huge ironies in gender roles are present all around us but usually go unnoticed. As I was exiting the hospital cafeteria one recent morning, a young woman approached the same door from the other side and opened it simultaneously with me. As often happens, an instant of confusion ensued regarding who was opening the door for whom. She conceded and passed through first, thus allowing me to be the one who had opened the door for her. I suppose a tiny remnant of chivalry, and perhaps inequality, persists.

In that instant, I was impressed by how familiar and unremarkable this little drama was in Western culture and, at the same time, how intolerable it would be in some cultures. This young woman is a co-worker and is on essentially equal social standing with me. She has the same right to pass through the door first and the same right to open the door for me. The decision is hers as much as it is mine. She is a free person, a full citizen. She is dressed in slacks and a simple blouse, presumably because it is the outfit she chose for the day. That decision is also hers. She is unmarried. She is walking to the cafeteria alone. She is employed in the profession of her choice, went to college to learn the job, works for her living, and supports herself. She is not confined to a life of reproductive services. These are all things that are disallowed in fundamentalist Muslim society and in many other reactionary cultures around the world, where women are still forbidden from working outside the home, driving a car, or leaving their homes without a male family member.

The Judeo-Christian and Islamic religions have divergent views on female human rights, and it is a major force driving their current conflict. When the United States entered the Afghanistan war, the rallying point focused on the Taliban's mistreatment of women. Images flashed across the TV screens, to be burned into our memories, of Taliban thugs beating women with nightsticks while the women cowered in their burkas. War widows begged in the streets for money to feed their starving children because they could not work or re-marry. According to their fundamentalist beliefs, the Taliban were fulfilling their responsibility to keep these women faithful to the will of Allah.

When the Ayatollah Khomeini called the United States "The Great Satan," he was referring to the lax morality of the Western culture. In Muslim culture, Satan is a seducer who corrupts others by setting a bad example. When fundamentalist Muslims look upon Western society, they respond the same way as the British upper class, who witnessed bare-breasted African native women. They see heathen barbarians. From the fundamentalist Muslim perspective, Western women walk around in public half-naked, exposing their bodies to every passing male without chaperones to secure their fidelity. They talk to any male they choose, spend time alone with whomever they choose, and engage in sex with whomever they choose. They display their sexuality publicly and use it to manipulate and influence the men around them. They work if they want, travel where they want, provide for themselves, and do as they please. The Sunni Muslim man wonders how faithful Muslim women can be expected to adhere to the moral standards revealed by Allah to his prophet, Muhammad, when they witness such immoral behavior among Western women. The answer, of course, is that they cannot. When given the opportunity, most Muslim women quickly abandon the restrictions of the fundamentalist Islamic culture.

The Western world offends fundamentalist Muslims not because of the actions of Western nations but rather because of the very existence of the Western culture. It is intolerable. The fundamentalist Muslims cannot live in peace with Westerners. Their religious beliefs, particularly those regarding the role of women, make peaceful co-existence impossible. The war between fundamentalist Muslims and the West, which is currently being fought worldwide, is the direct result of the difficulties human males incur in their efforts to control the reproductive choices of human females. Human sexuality has wide-ranging social, political, and military repercussions.

The Western world has seen tremendous upheaval in the past century. Wives are no longer the husbands' property but are of equal standing, legally and economically. Women are rapidly regaining the freedom and power they had before the invention of the plow and the domestication of cattle. The history of marriage over the past 5000 years has been a tale of the struggle between men and women over who controls the paternity of children. Western cultures are returning to the ancient ways in which the females choose which males reproduce, just as the peahens choose which peacocks reproduce. Perhaps this 5000-year-long nightmare for women is finally ending. As human females regain their sexual freedom, they will also regain control over which males fertilize their ova.

WHY IS IT SO HARD TO TALK ABOUT SEX?

Sex has probably been a sensitive subject of discussion since before the time of Homo sapiens. It is fraught with dangers, awash with competition and strife, and steeped in intrigue. There are good, basic reasons for being guarded and secretive about sex. It is unwise to divulge valuable information carelessly. Insights shared with a family member or neighbor may make that person a stronger competitor or even an enemy. Discretion in sexual matters is a basic human survival skill. This was not done out of shame but just out of caution and common sense. However, this basic instinct causes humans to be vulnerable to a method of control called shame.

The intrusion of religion into marriage created what we now think of as the nuclear family. It sanctified the male-female dyad and encouraged fidelity for both men and women. It has been a successful strategy, but there is a downside. The primary means of suppressing promiscuity was shame, applied liberally to any form of sexuality. It is still being applied today. Non-reproductive sex of any kind was once forbidden and is still considered hedonistic. Boys and girls are told from an early age that sex is sinful, unhealthy, and dangerous. They are shamed for their sexuality. They are shamed for masturbation. They are actively discouraged from exploring their bodies and their sexuality. Any sex education they receive is devoted to technical knowledge and the avoidance of pregnancy and disease. There are no instructions about how to achieve orgasm or how to acquire and retain a sexual partner. (Of course, the Internet has changed this drastically.)

The institution of shame continues into adulthood. Pornography is condemned. Prostitution is illegal. Premarital and extramarital sex are penalized. Public nudity is prohibited so fiercely that a mother cannot breastfeed her infant in public for fear of running afoul of morality laws. Talking about sex is forbidden in public places and the workplace. Jokes about sex are considered taboo. If told at work, they violate federal laws. The message delivered by religious and civil authorities to the people is consistent. Sex is evil, dangerous, and shameful except in the setting of a marriage sanctioned by authorities. People become so burdened by negative emotions about sex that they cannot enjoy or even discuss this most wonderful attribute of humanity.

Condemnation of sexuality is a two-edged sword. It is an effective tool for managing the reproductive behavior of a population. It reduces teen pregnancy, keeps adolescents in school, and encourages two-parent families and paternal investment in children. However, it creates a huge conflict between our natural feelings and the needs of modern society, and it prevents us from resolving those conflicts. Adolescents are too ashamed to ask parents or teachers meaningful questions about sex. Parents are too embarrassed and fearful to answer children's questions truthfully. Non-parent adults fear social and legal consequences if they answer adolescent sex questions too honestly. Suppression of sexuality has encouraged nuclear families and strengthened society but at a cost to the mental health of the population.

Many readers will find this book difficult to read simply because the subjects are so sensitive. But, if you have come this far, let us continue forward with courage. The next chapter covers material you have always wanted to know but were afraid to ask.

CHAPTER TEN
THE COMPLEX FEMALE ORGASM

When modern woman discovered orgasm, it was, combined with birth control, perhaps the biggest single nail in the coffin of male dominance.

— EVA FIGS

The last chapter considered men's struggle to control women's reproductive choices. This chapter explains why it is such a difficult task. Women are designed in a way that gives them a great deal of control over who fertilizes their ova.

The human female is a tough opponent. Her time of fertility is hidden and brief, but she is sexually active all through her monthly hormone cycle. She is genetically programmed to use her sexuality to obtain resources from many males while discreetly choosing which male will fertilize her egg. For the most part, this occurs without any awareness or effort on her part.

All human mating behavior, beginning with the first inquisitive eye contact, is part of a social dance that leads, if successful, to the act of sex. It is a complicated sorting process where males choose females and females choose males. However, the competition and selection do not stop when coitus begins.

The physiology of sex is complex, and a lot of activity is going on under the surface, literally and figuratively. While lovers are engaged in the mechanics of having sex, the internal genitalia are busy, too. The male focuses on delivering his gametes but also unwittingly performs other functions. The female is not just a passive receptacle for sperm. Her body can utilize the semen of different males selectively, based on her motives for having sex with them.

It can be difficult to decide just where to begin a discussion about copulation. A long chain of events leads up to sex. Lovers must first overcome the social hurdles and ego boundaries described in the previous chapters. This chapter begins when the lovers are disrobed, with their limbs intertwined, each trying to maneuver the other into a favorable position.

The male has a ready supply of sperm in his vas deferens, the tubes leading from the testicles. He has also generated a supply of seminal fluid in the prostate. His penis is engorged with blood, filling the various compartments until the longitudinal and circumferential strands of connective tissue are stretched tight, making the organ rigid. His heart rate and breathing rate are increased. All the muscles in his body are tense, and his senses are heightened. The primitive senses of touch, smell, and taste are amplified. His brain is focused on the feelings in his skin, especially on the mouth and genitalia, but also on his hands and all over his body.

In females, things are more complicated. Her physiology varies according to her hormonal state, which is dependent on her place in the menstrual cycle. Near ovulation, the female in estrus is more likely to be motivated by pleasure. At this point in her cycle, her mindset is much like that of the male, who is driven by simple lust. The female who is not in estrus may also feel lust, or she may have sex for ulterior motives unrelated to her pleasure. Unlike a male, the female can engage in intercourse when not aroused.

Assuming she is aroused, her genitalia are swollen and engorged, although not as obvious as the male. Both sexes have genital organs of the same basic design. The female has the same compartments engorged with blood as the male. He has the penis and its related structures, while she has the clitoris and its related structures, and both work the same way. Hers are smaller than his, but they are equally entertaining.

Her vagina is secreting a lubricating fluid from pores in the walls, wetting the entire internal surface. Her Bartholin's glands on the inner walls of the labia minora are secreting a white substance that looks and feels like a high-quality hand lotion. The labia majora and labia minora are swollen and separated. This opens the door of the vagina, allowing easy entrance for the penis.

If all goes well, as the lovers maneuver each other into position, he has no difficulty finding her vagina, and she has no difficulty admitting him. If he is uncircumcised, his foreskin will contact her labia, and his glans will easily slide through his foreskin and into the vaginal opening. If he is circumcised, he may meet some resistance when pushing the swollen glans past the labia unless he has allowed enough time for the Bartholin's glands to do their job thoroughly.

She flexes her hips and spreads her knees wide apart if they are in the missionary position. He spreads his knees apart and flexes his hips so that he supports his weight on his arms and knees, and his thighs push hers up and apart. She may put her legs behind him, clasping him and pulling him to her. He alternately advances and retracts his penis from her vagina. This stimulates the skin on his penis, the skin and mucosa of her labia, and the mucosa in the vagina, causing pleasurable sensations.

As their excitement mounts, he increases the speed and frequency of his thrusting into her vagina. He may have sudden involuntary thrusts, striking his mons pubis rather firmly against her vulva and striking her cervix with the end of his penis, causing rough movement of her internal pelvic organs. He may press himself firmly against her vulva, rocking his mons pubis against her external genitalia, especially the clitoris.

As she becomes more excited, she spreads her thighs wider and tilts her pelvis up. She rubs her genitals, especially her clitoris, against his mons pubis and the shaft of his penis. As she nears climax, her clitoris becomes hard and swollen. The firm clitoris may press against the sensitive dorsal surface of the base of his penis and stimulate him to climax. This can synchronize their orgasms.

If he is behind her, she may be standing, leaning over something, down on her elbows and knees (the knee-chest position), or even lying prone. She arches her lower back and pushes her buttocks back against him. If she is standing, she rises on her toes and tilts her pelvis backward, exposing her external genitalia rearward and giving him access to her vaginal opening. In this position, the male mons and penis do not contact the clitoris, and many women will not climax unless they stimulate the clitoris with their fingers.

However, some women favor this position for lovemaking. They have an exceptionally sensitive area in the front wall of the vagina, the G-spot, which will cause them to orgasm when it is stimulated. Rear entry rubs directly on this area.

MISCELLANEOUS POINTS OF INTEREST

This is a good place to digress and discuss a few frequently asked questions about human sexuality: penis size, foreskin, female ejaculation, and pubic hair. Penis size does matter, but not in the way most people think. Women vary remarkably in the size of their vaginas, and women with greater body fat have less accessible vaginas. Women with deep vaginas or heavy body habitus generally prefer men with longer penises. However, women who are thin or petite, have small vaginas or have sensitive pelvic interiors due to disease or scarring will prefer men with smaller penises. Likewise, women who have born children will prefer a larger diameter penis, while maidens or women who have had Cesarean births will prefer a smaller penis diameter. There is such a thing as too big, and it can be very uncomfortable for the woman. In the size of genitalia, as with everything else, the man and woman should be well-matched.

Some European historians believe that a mismatch in genitalia contributed to the French Revolution. King Louis XVI and Marie Antoinette were unable to produce an heir for the first eight years of their marriage because they could not engage in sex. Louis was endowed with a "bracquemart assez considerable," while Marie had "l'etroitesse du chemin." He had a large penis, and she had a small vagina, and they were unable to make love comfortably. The long delay in producing an heir prevented the formation of a strong military alliance between the Bourbons and the Hapsburgs, and the monarchy of France collapsed under the revolution.

The foreskin is another curious feature of human genital anatomy. Many mammals have a sheath of loose skin covering the penis. When the penis becomes erect, the sheath remains at the base. The human penile sheath is unique in that it is attached to the edge of the glans, far out toward the end of the penis. This is referred to as a foreskin, and in humans, it continues to cover part or all of the glans when the penis is erect. Even in males who have completely exposed glans on erection, the foreskin continues to fit loosely on the penile shaft.

It has been shown experimentally that this double layer of skin over the glans eases entry into an opening. The amount of force required to insert the tip of an erect penis into an orifice is reduced ten-fold by the presence of the foreskin over the glans. (Taves, 2002) The foreskin contacts the labia, and the glans slides through the foreskin, allowing easy entry into an unlubricated vagina. The loose skin on the shaft of the penis provides a glide function during coitus.

Most sex for primitive human females was not for pleasure but rather for ulterior motives (as it still is for women today). Sex generally occurs without the benefit of arousal and self-lubrication. The foreskin is an adaptation for sexual activity with an unaroused vagina. It is the male contribution to vaginal lubrication. Perhaps we would not need a personal lubricant industry if men were not circumcised.

Another point of interest is the G-spot. This is the location of the paraurethral gland around the urethra on the front wall of the vagina. The gland secretes fluid to moisten and lubricate the interior of the tube that leads from the bladder to the outside world. It is the equivalent of the prostate gland in males but much smaller. Like the prostate gland, it can be a source of pleasurable sensations when massaged. The size of the paraurethral gland is highly variable from one woman to the next. Some women have none, while others may be well endowed. Therefore, some women respond to stimulation of the G-spot, and others do not. It is also why some women enjoy rear-entry sex more than others.

A woman with a large paraurethral gland can eject a small amount of fluid at orgasm, just like the male ejects fluid from the prostate gland to produce semen. This is the source of the female ejaculate that some women produce. Individual variation in the size of the paraurethral gland is the reason some women ejaculate, and others do not.

Female ejaculation remains a controversial subject in modern literature, with many researchers denying that it occurs. However, astoundingly, many scientists and physicians thought the female orgasm was a myth until it was proven to exist in the 1960s by Masters and Johnson. The history of both female orgasm and female ejaculation goes back into antiquity. Aristotle (384 – 322 B.C.E.) discussed both phenomena, as did the Greek physician Galen of Pergamon (129 – 199 C.E.). In Muslim antiquity, according to Sahih al-Bukhari 3329 Book 60, Hadith 4, when Muhammad was asked what determines whether a child will look like the father or the mother, he responded, "If a man has sexual intercourse with his wife and gets discharge first, the child will resemble the father, and if a woman gets discharge first, the child will resemble her." The Hadith is the narrative of the life of Muhammad. It was written about 200 years after the death of Muhammad, so we have no way of knowing whether this record is historically accurate. However, the individual who recorded it knew human females sometimes have a liquid discharge at the climax of sexual intercourse.

Primitive people are also aware of the existence of the female orgasm. A !Kung San woman chastises a man who climaxes and then leaves her unsatisfied. If he does not complete his task, she will find someone who will. The unsatisfactory male may thus lose his opportunity to reproduce.

Finally, pubic hair serves several functions. Humans have lost almost all their body hair but retain hair in the armpits and over the genitalia. These are high-friction areas, and the hair serves as a dry lubricant. It prevents chafing. Pubic hair also provides visual cues to reproductive status. It is only present in reproductive-age people. Prepubescent children have no pubic hair, and postmenopausal women may lose the hair on their mons and genitals. In addition, the shape of the genital hair patch is different for men and women. The female escutcheon is a triangle pointed downward, and the male escutcheon is pointed upward due to an extension up the midline of the lower abdomen. When people are naked, this provides additional visual clues to a person's sex from a safe distance.

DURING THE CLIMAX

Returning to the act of copulation, other interesting things are happening. As the couple approaches orgasm, their genitalia become more engorged. The penis grows larger and firmer, and the glans swells. The scrotum contracts and pulls the testicles close against the body. The clitoris also swells, but just before orgasm, it retracts under the clitoral hood, perhaps to avoid injury.

If the female has semen left in her vaginal vault from sex with a prior male, her current lover removes it before he ejaculates. The shape of the glans on his penis, with its rounded point and flared rim, acts like a bilge pump, removing any fluid from the vagina. This occurs in both circumcised and uncircumcised men because thrusting into the vault retracts the foreskin. The human male with an adequately sized penis will remove his adversary's semen from a female's vagina. The previous male, who left the woman unsatisfied, thus loses his chance to reproduce. This mechanism favors the male with a larger diameter penis and explains why human males have the largest-diameter penis of all primates.

If the female is near ovulation, she has an ovulatory cyst on the surface of her ovary. The cyst is about one centimeter in diameter and contains a tiny ovum. Most women alternate right and left ovaries from month to month, but some women form ova in both ovaries every month, which is the most common cause of twins. As the ovum ripens, the fluid-filled chamber enlarges, and the cyst wall becomes thin and fragile.

When the ovum is mature, the cyst on the ovary waits patiently for several days. Eventually, it ruptures spontaneously, causing ovulation. When the cyst ruptures, the ovum is spilled out onto the fimbria, a patch of soft carpet-like tissue on the end of the fallopian tube. Sometimes, ovulation hurts, and some women can tell every month exactly when they have ovulated.

The ovum and the fluid in the cyst contain chemicals that attract sperm. When ovulation occurs, these chemicals diffuse outward and form a gradient or a trail for the sperm to follow to the ovum.

The rough jumbling of a woman's internal pelvic organs during copulation may rupture the ovulatory cyst, causing ovulation to occur during sex. The male who is engaged in sex with her at the time is then more likely to be the one to fertilize her ovum and impregnate her. He who has a long enough penis to rupture her ovulatory cyst has the best reproductive success. This is another reason the human male has a large penis.

The male climax consists of several stages, but the result is that the sperm in the vas deferens combines with the seminal fluid in the seminal vesicles and prostate. This mixture is propelled through the urethra by a series of peristaltic waves and is deposited in the vaginal vault near the cervix. At the same time, many other muscles in the pelvis and genitalia spasm rhythmically, and muscles of the back and limbs contract powerfully. The male experiences an overwhelming sensation of pleasure, and his oxytocin level immediately increases to five times the resting level.

The female climax is similar in many ways to that of the male. Her body responds in the same manner as his, with rhythmic spasms of the muscles in the pelvis and powerful contractions of the limb and back muscles. Her genital organs are also busy during orgasm. The vaginal opening contracts while the vault relaxes. The cervix and uterus undergo peristaltic waves, pumping semen to the fallopian tubes. Of course, she also experiences extreme pleasure with a fivefold increase in oxytocin.

Primitive people did not know these processes, and, for the most part, neither do modern humans. When people have sex, they are mostly in it for the oxytocin boost. If you ask individuals *why* they have sex, the most common answer given by men is, "Because it feels good." Women are more likely to answer, "Because he wanted to."

If everything goes right, the male's thrusting jostles the uterus and ovaries and ruptures the ovulatory cyst, releasing the ovum into the fimbria of the fallopian tube. The two lovers both have orgasms. The male ejaculates, depositing sperm and seminal fluid in the vagina near the cervix. The cervix and uterus draw up a small amount of semen and transport sperm up the fallopian tubes. Over the next ten minutes or so, the sperm swim the rest of the way to the fimbria, following the trail of chemical attractants secreted by the ovum. One sperm will penetrate and fertilize the ovum. The ovum membrane immediately seals itself, preventing any further sperm entry. The fallopian tube then transports the fertilized ovum to the uterus over several days. The developing embryo implants in the uterine wall and starts developing into a baby.

If the woman has an orgasm, her uterine contractions transport the sperm to the fallopian tubes by peristalsis. It is an active process on her part and a passive process on the part of the sperm. The sperm then swim the last few centimeters of the journey, following a trail of chemicals. This last part of the journey is a race. It selects for the swift and strong, leaving any defective sperm far behind and out of luck. If the woman has not had an orgasm, then the sperm are on their own to swim the entire distance from the cervix up the uterus, into the fallopian tubes, and up to the fimbria.

Of course, the great majority of copulations do not proceed in this fashion because most sex does not occur when the woman is ovulating. The human female is able to get pregnant for about twenty-four hours out of her twenty-eight-day menstrual cycle, but she can be sexually active for the entire twenty-eight days.

NON-REPRODUCTIVE SEX

The great majority of human sex is non-reproductive because it occurs when the woman is not ovulating or when she is pregnant, nursing, or postmenopausal. Most creatures do not have sex for any reason except to create offspring. Unlike most other animals, humans have sex for many reasons other than procreation. They have sex to pleasure themselves, pleasure each other, cement relationships, heal relationships after a rift, and reward their partners for various behaviors. Both men and women have sex for pure entertainment or to dominate each other; to trade for services, resources, or money; to obtain favorable social relationships or positions; to meet marital or religious obligations; to support their egos, heal their hurts, and distract themselves from other worries; and to stave off loneliness.

In their article, "Why Humans Have Sex," Cindy Meston and

David Buss identified 237 different reasons people gave for having their most recent episode of sex. The following table lists ninety of them.

<table>
<tr><td colspan="2">Why people have sex</td></tr>
<tr><td colspan="2">Here are some of the reasons for having sex given by college students, mostly single, ranging in age from 17 to 52 years of age. Adapted from Meston, Arch Sex Behav (2007) 36:477-507.</td></tr>
<tr><td>I was attracted to the person</td><td>It feels good</td></tr>
<tr><td>I wanted to experience the physical pleasure</td><td>I wanted to express my love</td></tr>
<tr><td>I wanted to show my affection</td><td>I was horny</td></tr>
<tr><td>I realized I was in love</td><td>I wanted to achieve an orgasm</td></tr>
<tr><td>I wanted to please my partner</td><td>The person's appearance turned me on</td></tr>
<tr><td>I wanted the pure pleasure</td><td>I was in the heat of the moment</td></tr>
<tr><td>It is exciting, adventurous</td><td>The person really desired me</td></tr>
<tr><td>The person caressed me</td><td>I wanted to feel connected to the person</td></tr>
<tr><td>I wanted to become one with the person</td><td>It was a romantic setting</td></tr>
<tr><td>I wanted to increase the emotional bond</td><td>The person made me feel sexy</td></tr>
<tr><td>The person was a good kisser</td><td>The opportunity presented itself</td></tr>
<tr><td>My hormones were out of control</td><td>I wanted to intensify the relationship</td></tr>
<tr><td>I wanted to feel loved</td><td>I wanted to reproduce</td></tr>
<tr><td>To celebrate a special event</td><td>I was curious about my sexual abilities</td></tr>
<tr><td>I was curious about sex</td><td>I was drunk</td></tr>
<tr><td>The person was intelligent</td><td>The person seemed self-confident</td></tr>
<tr><td>To keep my partner satisfied</td><td>I wanted to experiment</td></tr>
<tr><td>I wanted to improve my sexual skills</td><td>The person had beautiful eyes</td></tr>
<tr><td>I wanted to give someone an STD</td><td>I wanted to get a favor from someone</td></tr>
<tr><td>I wanted to get a raise</td><td>I wanted to punish myself</td></tr>
<tr><td>I wanted to get a job</td><td>It was a special occasion</td></tr>
<tr><td>The person offered me drugs for it</td><td>Someone offered me money to do it</td></tr>
<tr><td>I wanted to humiliate the person</td><td>I wanted to make money</td></tr>
<tr><td>I wanted to break up my relationship</td><td>I was angry</td></tr>
<tr><td>I wanted to be used or degraded</td><td>Because of a bet</td></tr>
<tr><td>I wanted to get a favor from someone</td><td>I wanted to get a promotion</td></tr>
<tr><td>It would get me gifts</td><td>I wanted to relieve menstrual cramps</td></tr>
<tr><td>It was a favor to someone</td><td>I wanted to get rid of a headache</td></tr>
<tr><td>To ruin rival's relationship via sex with his partner</td><td>To get revenge on partner who cheated</td></tr>
<tr><td>The person had lots of money</td><td>To gain access to that person's friend</td></tr>
<tr><td>I wanted to have more sex than my friends</td><td>I was physically forced to</td></tr>
<tr><td>I thought it would boost my social status</td><td>The person bought me jewelry</td></tr>
<tr><td>I wanted to stop my partner's nagging</td><td>My friends pressured me into it</td></tr>
<tr><td>I felt sorry for the person</td><td>To avoid hurting someone's feelings</td></tr>
<tr><td>I had not had sex in a long time</td><td>The person smelled nice</td></tr>
<tr><td>I am a sex addict</td><td>I thought it would relax me</td></tr>
<tr><td>So I could focus on other things</td><td>I wanted to act out a fantasy</td></tr>
<tr><td>The person was mysterious</td><td>An erotic movie had turned me on</td></tr>
<tr><td>I wanted to feel older</td><td>I wanted to feel closer to God</td></tr>
<tr><td>I wanted to keep warm</td><td>I thought it would help me fall asleep</td></tr>
<tr><td>I wanted to have a child</td><td>The person bought me an expensive dinner</td></tr>
<tr><td>I wanted to hurt an enemy</td><td>I wanted to reaffirm my sexual orientation</td></tr>
<tr><td>I was married and you are supposed to</td><td>I wanted to say "I'm sorry."</td></tr>
<tr><td>I wanted to feel younger</td><td>I wanted to make up after a fight</td></tr>
<tr><td>I was feeling lonely</td><td>I wanted to keep my partner happy</td></tr>
</table>

Most sex in humans is initiated by the male, who is relatively insensitive to the female's desires. Men want sex uniformly throughout the month. They do not have a hormone cycle. They are unaware of – or have only indirect clues to – when a woman is in estrus. Women can enjoy sex most of the month, but they feel the strongest physical urge to seek out a sex partner on those few days of the month when they are in estrus and near ovulation.

As a woman approaches ovulation and her ovum matures, the levels of the hormone estradiol rise in her bloodstream. Estradiol is the female equivalent of testosterone. It stimulates her libido and puts her in estrus. While it is elevated, she will have increased sex drive, a tendency to roam, and increased ease and frequency of orgasms. Estradiol causes a woman to seek out sex for her pleasure and search for an attractive opportunistic partner.

WHY WOMEN HAVE ORGASMS

The human female orgasm is an enigma. It is not necessary for reproduction. Women can get pregnant without orgasms. They can enjoy sex without orgasms. Men must have orgasms to deliver their ejaculate to the cervix, but women do not have to orgasm at all. Some researchers believe it is just a vestigial function some women retain because men have orgasms, in the same way that men have nipples because women need nipples for breastfeeding. That seems blatantly sexist, a remnant of the Victorian era when the female vagina was considered strictly a passive receptacle. Female organs are not passive, and the orgasm is not a vestigial shriveled organ like the male nipple. An orgasm is a highly complex process. Such functions are not retained unless they somehow increase reproductive success.

Many theories exist about the purpose of the female orgasm. They are all flawed because they begin by assuming there is only one function. In *The Case of the Female Orgasm*, Elizabeth Lloyd reviewed the arguments for and against twenty-one theories. She concluded

that orgasm in women is superfluous and is not necessary for reproduction. This is true, but it is not the same as saying that orgasm
does not serve a useful purpose.

To help sort this out, let us consider what we know about female
orgasms.

- Women like orgasms. Orgasms reward and encourage
  sex.
- Women are more able to orgasm during estrus when they
  are ovulating and can become pregnant.
- Women prefer a different, more masculine mate when
  they are in estrus. They choose men more for physical
  attraction.
- Women are more inclined to orgasm when they are more
  aroused.
- Women are more aroused by a partner they consider
  more attractive.
- Female orgasm transports sperm to the ovum in many
  mammals.
- Female orgasm stimulates ovulation in many mammals.
- Fluid transport by orgasm is very difficult to demonstrate
  experimentally in humans, but it has been shown in at
  least one study.
- A tiny amount of ejaculate transport during orgasm
  would greatly benefit the male who stimulated the
  woman to orgasm.

This strongly suggests that female orgasm plays a role in sexual
selection in humans. It allows a woman to subconsciously choose
which of multiple sexual partners will father her children.

Some women say they never have orgasms. Others say they
always have orgasms. Neither is true. Even the most non-sensual
woman, if she is healthy, will orgasm if she is given the proper

devoted attention by her Prince Charming (or Princess Charming). Likewise, even the most sensual woman will not orgasm during sex under conditions that are repulsive to her. The one indisputable fact about the female orgasm is that all women are selective about when and with whom they have orgasms. Women can choose whether to have an orgasm during a sexual liaison. They can choose whether to have sex for pleasure or for business.

A woman can unconsciously use her orgasm to select the father of her child. She is more inclined to search out a lover when she nears ovulation, and she is more likely to choose that sexual partner based on his attractiveness. Her elevated estradiol levels and his attractiveness make her more likely to orgasm with him and more likely to transport his sperm directly to the fallopian tubes at the time of ovulation. If his penis is large enough, and she is near ovulation, and the sex is energetic enough, he will rupture her ovulatory cyst during sex. Her orgasm will pump his semen to the ovum, and she will be pregnant about ten minutes after they climax.

A woman with sexual freedom may have sex with her proper mate ten times a month and with an illicit lover once a month, yet she is more likely to be impregnated by the lover. Of course, it is not a sure thing, but the man she chooses based on pure lust has a definite advantage. Meanwhile, she gets the best of both worlds. She gets all the social benefits she has accrued from having sex with her regular partner(s), and she still gets to choose the genetics of her offspring. The other males are none the wiser because they are completely unaware of her cycle. Every male who has copulated with her before her liaison with her lover or who copulates with her during and after her pregnancy may provide additional support to her and the child.

Returning to the matter of a woman's choice whether to orgasm during sex, imagine a male and female bargaining in a prehistoric tropical forest. Think of them as a negotiating pair. He has something she wants, and she has something he wants, but he is at a severe disadvantage in this parley. He does not know how much interest she has in his product or services. On the other hand, she knows exactly how much interest he has. She can see his penis. Furthermore, she can control his level of interest by enticing him, intruding on his personal space, or touching him. She knows he wants sex, and she can join him just for the pleasure, placing the two of them on an even playing field. Alternatively, she can choose not to pursue pleasure (or at least give him that impression) and instead trade for something else. She can barter for food, labor, protection, devotion, and the like. She gets a lot more in trade for her services if she keeps him in the dark about her desires.

Nature has given women so much power that the law has very wisely given them little.

— SAMUEL JOHNSON

Primitive women controlled men because they had a natural advantage. Their sexual desires were hidden from men, while men's desires were displayed openly. To use a poker analogy, women hold their cards close to the chest, while men's cards are on the table for all to see. This allowed women to obtain what they needed from men.

Recall that a mother needs support continually, not just when ovulating. If men could tell when a woman is in estrus and wanting sex, she would get male devotion for three days out of every two years (the average birthing cycle). On the other hand, if all women were orgasmic all the time, sex would be its own reward, and they would not get material rewards in return for sex. Women must keep men in the dark about how much they are interested, how much they are aroused, and when they are willing. That way, men who want sex from women are left with no other option but to keep knocking on the door with enticements and promises of devotion in expectation of occasional success. For women to get the most support from men, some must be highly interested in sex (easily orgasmic) and others completely disinterested (lesbians), with the majority scattered in between and constantly changing.

Researchers have been asking the wrong question. Instead of asking why women have orgasms, they should be asking why women vary so much in their ability to orgasm. It is the variability in female interest that ensures sustained support from men.

Incidentally, this answers another age-old question. "Why is it that men can never figure out what women want?" It is because male ignorance best serves the needs of women and their children.

Of course, most modern human females are not so promiscuous and do not rely on multiple men for their support. Today, the paternity of most children is known. However, the anatomy and physiology in humans today originated when human reproduction was chaotic and highly promiscuous. The genes that drive human instincts today are the same genes that survived and prospered in Paleolithic times. Sexual drives have not changed.

Paternity is now easily detectable using DNA analysis. A study in England revealed that one out of every 400 sets of fraternal twins was fathered by two different men. This means one out of every 400 women with fraternal twins was inseminated by two different men within three days. Of course, women who bear fraternal twins are no different morally or ethically from women who bear single infants. Therefore, the researchers concluded one out of every four hundred pregnancies in England is of uncertain paternity because the woman's fallopian tubes contained sperm from two or more men when she was ovulating.

Another study, also in England, asked married women whether they had been inseminated by two men within a thirty-minute time interval at any time in their lives. One out of every two hundred women said they had. When the time interval was twenty-four hours, thirty percent responded affirmatively. When the time was three days, seventy percent said yes. Sperm usually survive for three days inside a woman. This means seventy out of every hundred women in the study group had risked a pregnancy of uncertain paternity at some time in their lives.

In England, a modern industrialized nation dominated by Judeo-Christian cultures, the level of promiscuity is high enough to generate competition between the sperm of different males inside the pelvis of most females at some time in their lives. In that kind of competitive setting, any advantage is significant. The male who stimulates the female to orgasm has a considerable edge over the male who does not. She assists his sperm in reaching her ovum and impregnating her. Even if the pregnancy does not happen on this occasion, this male has the right combination of personality and genital anatomy that works for her. She is more likely to choose him a month later when she again looks for a lover.

The female orgasm has far-ranging social and political implications. When men first tried to seize control of paternity 5000 years ago, this is what they were up against. Women choose the father of a child in a manner completely mysterious to men. They selectively transport the sperm from their chosen lover to their ovaries. In trying to control the paternity of women's offspring, men were defying the natural order of things. They were attempting to deprive women of the female role in sexual selection. In their ignorance and determination, men committed – and are still committing – a host of human-rights violations. These reveal the insecurity husbands feel in the face of their chief adversaries – their wives.

OTHER POSSIBLE ROLES OF THE FEMALE ORGASM

Many people believe that female orgasm encourages women to have sex and have children. There are problems with this line of logic. Women have sex and get pregnant in the absence of orgasms. Ten to twenty percent of women never have orgasms during sex with men. Many women who orgasm during sex do so by self-manipulating the clitoris (assisted coitus). That is, they masturbate while having sex with a man. Only about twenty percent of women reliably have orgasms during unassisted coitus. This is not a very effective device for rewarding women to have sex.

Orgasm for women during unassisted coitus requires much longer (an average of twenty minutes) than orgasm by self-stimulation (an average of four minutes). Women who do not orgasm at all with men still orgasm by masturbation with the same success rate as other women. Women achieve orgasm through clitoral stimulation in about the same time it takes men to achieve orgasm through coitus or masturbation, that is, in about four minutes. So the only time women take longer than men to orgasm is when they have sex with men. It seems the orgasm may encourage women to have sex, <u>but not with men</u>.

Women who can form strong emotional bonds with other women have an additional option available when searching for assistance in raising their offspring. Human females need help raising their young, but it does not have to come from males. One of the functions of the female orgasm may be to encourage human females to engage in sex not with males but with females. All evidence indicates human females achieve orgasm more easily during masturbation than during sex with males. Perhaps the female orgasm is more important to homosexual sex than heterosexual coitus. If so, it provides women with an alternative, safer means of obtaining the support they need during pregnancy and nursing. Maybe women were not intended to orgasm with men, except with Mr. Right during ovulation. Perhaps most orgasms were with other females.

Consider the advantage of Paleolithic females who had a powerful tool for cementing social bonds between themselves without the males. In the primitive setting, a single male could dominate a single female, but a coalition of females could overpower an abusive or oppressive male. This pattern has been well documented among female bonobos, who routinely use homosexual sex to form coalitions. Subsequently, they use those coalitions to dominate the males and control the social structure of the troop. I suspect human females once did likewise.

Paradoxically, the human trait that makes men so easy to exploit, the extreme male sex drive, also makes men annoying and often dangerous. The most common complaint from wives is that their husbands want too much sex. Men pester women for sex, and quarrels about sex are ubiquitous in marriages. Men have instincts that drive them to force women into sex. The human male brain is focused on obtaining sex with women by whatever means available. Lone women fear men. A woman feels much safer in a crowd.

It is intriguing to rethink the dioecious family structure in this context. Perhaps this is why so many indigenous cultures adopted separate housing for men and women. A group of women can hold their own against individual men. Sex between women is a powerful device for binding a group of women together. This topic will be explored in greater depth in the section on sexual diversity.

ONE MORE CONSIDERATION

During the Stone Age, sex was not restricted by laws and religion, and female sexuality was not suppressed. It may be that under primitive conditions of high promiscuity, many more females were orgasmic. If Laumann et al. (1994) are correct, and the average American female has only six sexual partners in a lifetime, then many women may not experience enough partners to find one with the precise combination of personality, coital pattern, and genital anatomy to induce orgasms. Maybe modern women have low rates of coital orgasm because modern cultures restrict their opportunities to sample enough lovers.

The Abrahamic religions have rigidly suppressed female sexuality. Girls are taught that sex is bad and that their sexual desires are abnormal and shameful. They are admonished to avoid any sexuality, including masturbation. Young women are deprived of any opportunity to learn how to orgasm. I suspect women would be a great deal more orgasmic if they did not have so much oppressive moral guidance in their youth. That oppression, of course, is the heart of the matter. From an early age, women are discouraged from enjoying sex because men want to control the paternity of children.

> Come out Virginia, don't let 'em wait. You Catholic
> girls start much too late.

— BILLY JOEL

CHAPTER ELEVEN

FINDING EACH OTHER

I was looking for love in all the wrong places
Looking for love in too many faces

— WANDA MALLETTE, BOB MORRISON,
AND PATTI RYAN

Laumann (1994) offers three useful models of the social tools people use to locate and assess prospective mates: social networks, economic choices, and cultural scripts. Before these can be initiated, though, a single person must have some idea of what they are searching for.

The most difficult part of choosing a mate often lies in each person deciding what he or she wants. Most people simply do not know. They are much better at identifying what they do not want. They have a vague template of an ideal mate constructed from relationships with parents, religious instructions, traditional narratives, fairy tales, peer pressure, and television. People wander around, sampling each other, comparing them to the templates, and discarding those who do not match. For the most part, people are not aware of the templates and do not know what they are seeking. However, both men and women have certain genetically programmed desires, certain instincts.

Men instinctively search for both long-term and short-term mating opportunities and have vastly different criteria for the two types of mates. For a man, a potential long-term mate is a woman with good parenting potential, a high degree of fidelity, social network compatibility, and the right attractiveness. A man instinctively looks for youth, good health, symmetric features, and the hourglass figure.

A potential short-term mate is almost any woman who is available for sex. A male may gain additional progeny from every opportunity for coitus with any female, with no further investment on his part. The emphasis is on availability, with only secondary concerns for attractiveness, health, and safety.

Women also instinctively search for both long-term and short-term mating opportunities. A woman instinctively searches for a long-term mate who will be a good provider. She judges a man in terms of his employment (formerly his hunting skills), resources, quality of clothing and automobile, and his social rank among other men. She also looks for a man who can provide physical protection and prefers someone in good health and good physical shape.

In a long-term mate, a woman instinctively prefers a frugal man. She does not want someone who throws away resources she may one day consider to be hers. This contrasts with a woman's short-term strategy, when she looks for a man who easily gives away money or resources. The primitive short-term strategy is directed mostly toward obtaining resources – she wants a man to spend money on her with few expectations in return.

Short-term mating instincts in the human female may have an alternative goal. A woman who already has a long-term partner can obtain a higher quality of genetic material for her offspring from a short-term partner. This strategy compels her to seek discreet opportunistic couplings with highly attractive males during her fertile period. If she is in estrus and the proper opportunity arises, she has an instinctive drive to aggressively pursue sex with a male of high physical attractiveness, bravado, or political power.

That summarizes, in a very condensed fashion, the instincts driving people in their search for mates, based on their genetic programming. Fulfilling those desires is another matter.

SOCIAL NETWORKS

Your social network is the collection of all the people you know and all the people they know. For mating purposes, it is everyone who is aware you are available and searching for a mate.

Social networks are complex, real-life communication networks. A special branch of mathematics is dedicated to the subject, and when applied to matching applications, it is called social-network analysis. It is widely used in computerized matchmaking and other Internet applications, such as targeted advertising and Facebook. Internet applications allow users to join virtual social networks that link users according to their relationships. Users can graphically visualize their entire social networks through figures displaying connecting points and lines between members. These Internet utilities are highly simplified. Real-life social networks are much more complicated and much less transparent.

Everyone has a social network. It includes co-workers, clients, vendors, supervisors, family, extended family, in-laws, casual acquaintances, and members of one's church and sports teams. School adds a network of classmates, teachers, the classmates of one's children, the parents of those children, and alumni. Most people have primary social networks containing hundreds of people, with each of those people having their own social network. The extended social network of an average person typically contains thousands of people.

The great majority of people in the social network are not potential mates due to age, sex, sexual preference, religion, social standing, social connections, attractiveness, or availability. There are many exclusions. Humans do not date their kin. Medical-care workers do not date their patients or family members of the patients. Supervisors do not date subordinates. People generally prefer mates close to their age. Hindus do not date Muslims, who do not date Jews. Fundamentalist Christians do not date atheists. Highly educated women do not date uneducated men, and low-earning men do not attempt to woo high-earning women. The list goes on and on. The first task is to identify those few individuals who have some reasonable chance of being contenders. The role of a good social network is to find candidates, sort them out, identify potential mates, and bring them together.

Consider potential mates identified in a social network in the following manners. Two people choose each other from among acquaintances drinking at the same bar. All they know about each other is they are both lonely and drink alcohol. That is not very promising. If they choose each other from among co-workers at their place of employment, at least they know they both have jobs. They also have some idea of each other's social standing and level of education.

When two people meet through their church activities, they have more in common. They know each other's ethical frameworks, religious beliefs, and social standing in the community. They also share their social networks and personal values. The information they receive is somewhat reliable.

If two people are introduced by their mothers, chances are the information they receive about each other is based on the mothers' wishes rather than on the truth. It is not very reliable. An introduction by one's sibling has greater potential to identify a possible mate. An introduction by a roommate is even better. A roommate is more likely to know a person's true habits and idiosyncrasies and what they want in a potential mate.

The social network filters potential mates through a process in which the network members make decisions on behalf of an individual. Friends and acquaintances decide who should and should not be encouraged. An individual actively searching for a mate makes the fact known to the social network. The members of the network then initiate networking. Human beings are natural-born matchmakers.

Of course, there will be many disagreements within the network. Full consensus is rare. Members have competing goals, and individuals may have hidden agendas. Jealousy, spite, and intrigue can muddle the network filtering process. Ultimately, in a free society, individuals seeking mates must make decisions for themselves.

That is not true in all cultures. Over the past five thousand years, most marriages have been arranged, even in the Judeo-Christian cultures. Recall, this was the theme of *Fiddler on the Roof*. According to the Russian Jews' tradition, a matchmaker in the community would choose spouses for young adults; without such traditions, people would be as precarious as a fiddler on the roof.

Some cultures today still allow members of the social network to make mating decisions. Most traditional Hindu marriages are arranged, and many Hindu couples do not meet each other until a few days before their wedding. Family members and professional matchmakers perform all searches and selections and make most mating decisions. The wedding participants have little opportunity for input. In conservative Muslim societies, women are confined to residences and have no opportunity to find or choose mates. Their social networks, comprised of relatives and acquaintances, choose their prospective mates. However, Muslim women do have some say in the decision. Sharia Law allows Muslim women to veto a proposed marriage. A Muslim woman and her male guardian must approve of a potential husband before the marriage can occur.

THE ECONOMIC MODEL

In Western societies, men and women are now free to make reproductive choices. They do not suffer the oppression (or enjoy the luxury) of proxy decision-makers. They must weigh the opportunities and the risks and decide for themselves. One paradigm for decision making is based on economics and individual social capital.

Social capital encompasses all the things your social network projects onto you that determine the net value of your persona. It can be viewed as a group of commodities. That is to say, you own your social capital. It consists of such things as your self-esteem, reputation, time, wealth, youth, beauty, health, personal safety, freedom, legal standing, earning potential, reproductive potential, social rank, and education. You can envision social capital as the stuff that flows back and forth within the social network. These are the things you have to offer to another person.

Every interaction people have with their social network requires some social capital investment. It places something at risk and promises a return on that investment. Proposing a new idea at work is a notoriously risky business with a high potential for gain or loss. Giving a speech or a toast at a public event is a chance to shine, or an opportunity for humiliation. Inviting someone to lunch is an investment intended to enhance a social bond, but it can also lead to rejection and loss of self-esteem. Going out on a date is an investment of time and money in hopes of building a relationship or enhancing one's social standing, but it places all that capital at risk if the date goes poorly.

A simple introduction involves the risk of rejection due to a botched name or a flubbed handshake. Every man knows the risk of a self-introduction to a woman. An entire branch of social science is dedicated to the subject of "pick-up" lines and the associated "get lost" responses. A Google search of "science of dating" + "pick-up lines" yields five thousand hits. Whole books are published on this one subject. It is all very anxiety-provoking. One risks the loss of self-esteem when using a pick-up line, but it is worth the risk if it may lead to an opportunity to reproduce. Personal choices are often made based on risk and benefit assessments, but people are generally not aware of the economic nature of their decisions.

Both men and women are very aware of the appearance of the

people with whom they are seen in public. Women want to show off a date who is "hot," while men like to be seen with "arm candy." Such public displays enhance their reputations and increase their social capital. The converse is true as well. A well-to-do woman will not want to be seen cuddling in public with a man dressed like a bum. A well-to-do man will not be pleased with his wife if she shows up at a public function with unkempt hair and no makeup.

Parents are certainly aware of this. They constantly worry about the company their children keep and the effects on their reputations. Reputation is an important part of social capital. A bad reputation closes doors and severs connections in one's social network. The value of reputation as social capital is evident when people speak of "loss of reputation" as if it were a physical entity.

Consider a woman who has been asked out on a first date by a man. She must decide whether she will benefit from a relationship with him. If she invests herself in this person, will she yield a return on that investment? Before she decides, she will need the answers to a long list of questions:

- What is his reputation, and will it enhance or tarnish hers?
- What is his potential as a long-term mate, based on earning power and education?
- How physically attractive is he?
- Would she want to be seen in public with him?
- Would she want her children to resemble him?
- Is he fun to be with?
- Does he have money, and is he willing to spend it on her?
- Would a long-term relationship with him enhance her wealth?
- Is he safe to be with? Does he have a history of violence, and would he harm her?

- Does he engage in criminal activity or substance abuse? Would he cause her to end up in jail or lose her earning potential?
- If she has children, how will he behave toward them? Will he accept them and father them, or will he be a risk to them?
- What are his intentions? Does he have a history of short-term relationships – just casual sex – or is he looking for a wife?

All this must be determined before she ever gets the chance to find out if she likes him. The members of her social network will be her sources of information. They will answer most of these questions for her.

Of course, the information she gets may not be reliable. Some members of her social network may be her adversaries who wish to sabotage the potential relationship. It is common for women to provide misleading information about eligible men. One woman may tell another that a man overstates his financial situation or employment prospects or that he is a philanderer. Members of her social network who are adversaries may also provide false information to the man, telling him she sleeps around, or, conversely, she does not give sex, depending on what the informant thinks the man is looking for in this woman.

The rules of fair play do not apply in love and war.

— JOHN LYLY, *EUPHUES* (1578).

The same is true for a man deciding whether to engage in or continue a relationship with a woman. He bases his initial decisions on information provided by his social network. He may solicit information from his male and female friends regarding her availability, and will receive unsolicited information as well. His mother will certainly have some input when she finds out about it.

The information he receives may be unwelcome, unverifiable, or untrue. He may have adversaries who seek her attention, and she may have adversaries seeking him. The most detrimental charge against a woman is promiscuity, leading a man to believe she will engage in infidelity. Other common derogatory assertions are that she stops giving sex after marriage or she wastes money or resources.

The economic model says every decision about relationships is made based on a risk-benefit assessment. A person must consider the potential risks and benefits of their options, knowing that assessments of both may be based on inaccurate or false information. Ultimately, each person, using the available information, must decide for himself or herself what to do next and whether to "sit it out or dance."

SCRIPTING

When a person chooses a course of action, he or she relies on knowledge of how other humans have acted in that situation. Every person carries a collection of memories gained from experiences, observations, live theater, movies, books, parents, oral traditions, and religious teachings. This amounts to a huge repertoire of scripts for social behaviors in every conceivable situation. Social-scripting theory suggests that people choose from these scripts when deciding how to act. That is, they are acting out a part they have seen elsewhere. They are following the examples set by their role models.

Human sexual responses are controlled by primitive instincts resulting from genetic programming, and they do not change from one generation to the next or from one culture to another. They are automatic behaviors left over from the Stone Age and are no longer appropriate in our modern world. Scripts, on the other hand, vary from one culture or generation to another. They depend on age, religion, legal climate, local customs, personal morals, and past experiences. Unlike other animals, humans can choose whether and how to act upon their instinctive urges. They get to choose which scripts to follow.

When an American woman dresses up, puts on her make-up, and goes out to a bar to attract men, she follows a script. She has arranged herself to draw the attention of males, inviting them to approach her. This allows her to reject all but the one she prefers. It is as if she were wearing a T-shirt that says on the front, "Please love me," and on the back, "No, not you."

When Hindu newlyweds, who have only known each other for a few days, engage in the first sex of their lives, they follow a script. When a father gives away his daughter to the groom in a Christian wedding, all three follow a script. It is usually part of a play they have rehearsed the prior evening.

The couple who elopes against the wishes of their parents is following a script called, "We are young and in love, and that is all that matters." When a wealthy older man marries a younger single mother and rescues her and her children from economic woes, he follows a script called "The White Knight." She is following a script called "My Prince." Pickup lines men and women use in bars, libraries, laundromats, and supermarkets are scripts. Rejection lines are also scripts. Both are rehearsed regularly.

Here is a description of a standard Western dating script:

"There are three possible parts to a date, of which at least two must be offered: entertainment, food, and affection. It is customary to begin a series of dates with a great deal of entertainment, a moderate amount of food, and the merest suggestion of affection. As the amount of affection increases, the entertainment can be reduced proportionately. When affection *is* the entertainment, we no longer call it dating. Under no circumstances can the food be omitted."

— MISS MANNERS' GUIDE TO EXCRUCIATINGLY

CORRECT BEHAVIOR BY JUDITH MARTIN

The rules of dating are scripts and vary in different cultures. In the Western urban culture, the standard script involves a male asking a female to attend an event with him, such as a dinner, concert, or party. He should ask her a minimum number of days in advance. Otherwise, he risks she will not accept the offer, either because she already committed her time to someone else or because she will not admit she does not already have a date for that evening. He pays her expenses for the evening and provides transportation.

On the initial date, they will go to a public place. They will both dress stylishly. They will talk about non-sexual matters and engage in non-sexual touching. Subsequent dates will become gradually more intimate until the couple finds themselves in the script depicted in the first few paragraphs of Chapter 10.

The modern world offers an endless variety of courting scripts. The young lovers who defy their social networks and end in disaster are like those depicted in *Pyramus and Thisbe, Romeo and Juliet, West Side Story*, and probably *The Graduate*, though the story ends prematurely. Since the beginning of time, damsels in distress have been rescued by their knights and princes. Powerful men have fallen from grace under the influence of their hormones and sensual women, from Helen of Troy to Monica Lewinski. Of course, the classic script everyone hopes to follow in the Western world is called "Happily ever after." The actors fall deeply in love, overcome all obstacles, and remain in romantic bliss until the end of time. Nevertheless, it is, after all, just a script, an act, a play. It is not real.

The acceptable scripts for modern dating in Western cultures can be found in a cornucopia of self-help books lining the shelves in Barnes and Nobles. The classic is *The Rules*, by Ellen Fein and Sherrie Schneider, which gives females the guidelines on finding and snaring Mr. Right. On the same shelf is a tongue-in-cheek male response entitled *The Code*, by Nate Penn and Lawrence LaRose, which tells males how to avoid being snared while still getting sexual access to females. Thousands of titles in between analyze fine details of dating, from the beginner's *Dating for Dummies*, by Joy Browne, to the advanced *Guerilla Dating Tactics*, by Sharyn Wolf.

The process of finding a mate was simple in prehistoric times. People lived in small groups and had small social networks. Humans are still genetically programmed for that time but now live in a completely different environment. The changes started with the development of towns and cities, sped up with long-distance transportation, and exploded with long-distance communication. Humans are designed to interact face-to-face with a few hundred individuals at most, only with as many people as live in a tribe or a few villages. Today, we are exposed to millions of people, mostly at a distance, via radio, television, telephone, the Internet, social networking, instant messaging, cell phones, and text messaging. It should not be surprising that our basic instincts feel dysfunctional.

People still find each other, though, ferreting out a signal in the cacophony of background noise. They still form couples and manage to spend enough time together to see if their ego boundaries collapse. They somehow learn enough about each other to determine whether there is a script they can share. Then they try to stay on the same page together long enough to form a pair bond and make a life and family together, usually without ever considering why.

CHAPTER TWELVE
AN ALARMING NOVELTY

Birth control is the first important step a woman must take toward the goal of her freedom. It is the first step she must take to be man's equal. It is the first step they must both take toward human emancipation.

— MARGARET SANGER

A woman needs a man like a fish needs a bicycle.

— IRMA DUNN

As the family goes, so goes the nation and so goes the whole world in which we live.

— POPE JOHN PAUL II

The end of the human race will be that it will eventually die of civilization.

— RALPH WALDO EMERSON

In the year 2525, if man is still alive, if woman can survive, they may find...

— RICK EVANS

We, as a species, are in the midst of great turmoil. Recall the remark by Somerset Maugham that the purpose of falling in love is to trick people into having children. When reproduction is separated from falling in love, it drastically alters the natural course of human history. The Law of Unintended Consequences states, "Intervention in a complex system always creates unanticipated and often undesirable outcomes." Let us now consider some unintended consequences of the ongoing changes in human sexual strategies.

We entered the modern age of human sexuality about 5000 years ago, coinciding with the suppression of female sexuality. Women rebelled about 100 years ago and began to regain their rights. Cultural change has snowballed in the past 50 years. Availability of effective birth control and reliable latex condoms have made it possible for both men and women to seek out short-term partners just for pleasure, with little concern for pregnancy or disease. Women have regained much of the sexual freedom they had in the Paleolithic era, and men have regained liberal sexual access to women. With economic equality, women can now make mating decisions without regard to the earning power of men, and men can obtain sex from women without incurring the expense of children.

Contraceptive technology has enabled the emergence of an entirely new class of humans. Their lifestyle has become so commonplace in the Western culture it is no longer recognized as a novelty. A huge segment of the population is now free from the burdens of child rearing while still enjoying their sexuality. Hundreds of millions of people can now expend their life efforts on whatever they choose, whether it is the advancement of human culture and science or simply the pursuits of leisure.

Look again at Dan and Alicia, who lived together through graduate school but separated in their professional lives. They completed their degrees and remained free of children when their pair bond ended. This would not have been possible as little as fifty years ago. Without birth control, they would have had children during their four years together, and those children would have constrained their professional and personal choices.

Birth control violates the assertion in the Book of Ecclesiastes that there is nothing new under the sun. When two healthy, reproductively mature mammals form a pair with some purpose other than creating offspring, this is genuinely new in the animal kingdom and truly a new thing under our sun. In fact, this is drastically, astoundingly, perhaps catastrophically new, and the possible consequences warrant scrutiny.

When women are financially independent of men, marriage and the traditional nuclear family become marginalized. When certain groups selectively adopt birth control, this non-uniformity changes the composition of the human gene pool. When men and women are near each other in the workplace, they must suppress their natural sexual behaviors. When the ratio of childless people to child rearing people increases drastically, it effectively de-thrones the clergy, the sterile caste, who have historically provided moral guidance and leadership to the reproductive population.

THE MARGINALIZATION OF MARRIAGE

Like Dan and Alicia, the great majority of childless adults are in relationships but not married simply because marriage has become superfluous. These are the childless-by-choice couples. Birth control, preventive medicine, civil engineering, and agriculture have made their existence possible. Birth control allows them to have a sexual relationship without the burden of children. They live in a land of plenty, with good health and ample food. When free of disease, famine, and war, they are not compelled to produce ten children so that two might survive. They do not need children to help them in the garden, farm, or family industry or business. They can put off having children or choose not to have them at all.

Birth control and economic equality have given women freedom – or rather given women back their freedom – to explore and exploit their sexuality. However, on the downside, when women can make themselves available to men without risk of pregnancy or need for support, men have access to casual sex with those women at a greatly reduced social cost to themselves. Increased sexual freedom for women also increases sexual access for men and, consequently, decreases sexual bargaining power for women. "Why buy a cow when you can get the milk for free?" Female control over access to the vagina and womb has historically been women's source of financial power. For eons, women have been able to obtain resources and commitments from men in exchange for the opportunity to reproduce using the women's bodies.

Many women are now self-sufficient, able to raise children without the support of a spouse. When women can go it alone, and so many are willing to do so, it becomes much more difficult for traditionally-minded women to recruit and retain husbands who would support them and their children in the long term. The bargaining power granted to chaste women by virtue of their possession of a womb is greatly reduced because their competitors have undersold them. The product they have to offer on the market has been devalued.

Add the Internet into the equation and traditionally-minded women do not stand a chance at securing mates in an old-fashioned way, offering their sexuality with strings attached. Out of eight billion websites on the Internet, four percent are pornographic. The Internet contains more photos and videos of naked women than there are women on Earth. At virtually zero cost, a man can have access to more women than he could use in a hundred lifetimes.

The value of male sex, on the other hand, has always been zero because men are willing to give it away freely. Men lose nothing and gain a great deal when sex becomes more available to all. However, from a reproductive point of view, the value of the sex men obtain from women is greatly diminished. Sex does not result in offspring when women use birth control or when the women are electronic images on a computer screen. Men have more access to women for sex but not for reproductive purposes.

It has become more difficult for young men to reproduce simply because young women are all using birth control. Women have always borne the greatest share of the burden of child rearing and are the most incentivized to avoid pregnancy. Independent young women make their own reproductive choices, disregarding young men's expectations.

Men contribute to a relationship, but their contributions have also been devalued. Men who want to raise a family have no leverage to obtain reproductive services from financially independent women on birth control. Such women no longer need the protection and provisions men once provided. Liberated women do not have to obligate themselves to a lifetime of child rearing to secure their futures.

My friend Alexis is now twenty-seven and unmarried. She was once in love with a young man her age. They went through college together and then parted. When I first met her years ago, she wanted six children. Now, she has no man in her life. She is well educated, friendly, pretty, and very bright. She looks like a woman who would have no trouble finding a mate. Alexis recently purchased her own home. She said it would be a nice place to raise children if she ever married, but she has not found anyone. It is difficult for a woman like Alexis to find a suitable mate, a man who would meet her emotional and intellectual needs and have higher earning power than she has. Alexis already has a home and a good income. Most men will not woo women like Alexis. They instead pursue women who have greater need for the services they bring to a relationship.

I suspect Alexis has defaulted into a matrilineal lifestyle, in which she needs a male only to father her children. When a man comes into her life, he will stay in her home only for the pair bond duration. They may not marry at all. When the romance fades, he will be left with no power base in the relationship. She will end the relationship and choose another man to replace him. As happens in primitive hoe-based agricultural societies, she will own the home, and the children. The men in her life will be transient.

This is the route my junior colleague Caroline has now taken. As a professional, she can support herself and her child without the assistance of a mate. She is free to leave her husband and be independent. She will survive just fine as a single mother. She does not need to be subservient to a male in return for his support. If she wants more children, she can choose another mate for that purpose.

Perhaps this is the underlying cause of the 2006 National Vital Statistics Report findings that the percentage of children born out of wedlock rose from twenty-nine percent to thirty-eight percent, even though the number of out-of-wedlock pregnancies among teenagers decreased. The increase was noted among women in their twenties and thirties who had children out of wedlock by choice.

Many independent women simply do not feel it is worth the trouble to have men in their lives, even after they have children. There often is no place for men in our modern, urban, civilized society. A man to a woman is like a bicycle to a fish. However, any woman who has ever had to remove a snake from the bathroom, free up a farm tractor from four feet of mud, clear a fallen tree from the road, or simply change a flat tire on the roadside, quickly learns to appreciate the value of a man. There are still times when men are very useful.

The Western world is now civilized. The wolves, hyenas, and snakes are gone from suburbia. The roads and bridges are all built. Food comes from the local grocery store. What is there for a man to do in daily life that a woman cannot? The answer, of course, is that a man can impregnate a woman. An independent woman needs nothing else from the father of her child she cannot obtain on her own or from other women.

This is a drastic change from one hundred years ago. Women

needed men for support, and when women needed men, they had sex with men, and they ended up having babies. However, when women are independent of men, they have fewer offspring simply because they are not obligated to have sex without birth control. Bright, independent young women have fewer offspring compared to dependent women. They have lower reproductive success.

The Law of Unintended Consequences
An Illustration

All unwed pregnant women in the U.S. are automatically eligible for Medicaid benefits. The government will pay all the costs of the pregnancy, delivery, and post-partum care for an unmarried woman. As a result, it has become commonplace for uninsured couples to delay marriage until after they have a family.

But this behavior is not restricted to the poor. A local well-to-do attorney and business owner delayed marrying his live-in girlfriend until she delivered their second child. It was a simple business decision. Her medical bills were covered by tax dollars.

She is now among those women counted on the census as unwed mothers. The increased rate of childbirth to unwed mothers in their twenties and thirties is in part due to financial incentives from the government.

AN INTERESTING ENCOUNTER WITH TWO WOMEN

Connie, a twenty-six-year-old white female, came to my ER with low abdominal pain, which started during the night after she used intravenous crystal meth. Crystal meth does not generally cause abdominal pain, so I considered what else might have caused the patient's pain. Mostly, I thought about what she might have done to pay for the drugs she had consumed during the night. I asked one of my female ER techs, Vicky, to come with me as a chaperone while I interviewed and examined the patient. Vicky is a twenty-nine-year-old white female, a nursing student, and a professional secretary in the ER.

When I entered the exam room, I was surprised by how similar the two women looked. They were attractive and fresh-looking, with good complexions, symmetric features, and oval faces. They both looked like healthy, pretty farm girls.

I questioned the patient about her symptoms and the circumstances of her drug use. She had broad lower abdominal pain, and it hurt when she walked. She denied any pain with urination. She thought she might have a vaginal discharge. She had no nausea or vomiting. Her menses had been normal. A physician recently told her that she had a urinary tract infection and prescribed antibiotics and pain pills. She did not take the antibiotics, but she did take the pain pills.

She admitted she was unemployed and had no means of supporting herself. She had to "hustle" the drugs wherever she could. She admitted to prostitution in the past but claimed she had not done so in the last month. She admitted she did not have any money to pay for the drugs she had used during the night. She said she could not remember if she had sex during the night, but if she did, it was "non-consensual."

On examination, she had no abdominal tenderness. She also had no vaginal discharge and no internal tenderness on the pelvic exam. There were no wounds or bruises on her genitalia to indicate rape. Her urinalysis and pregnancy test were normal. I did not find any infection. I gave her a prescription for some mild pain pills and discharged her.

During the exam, I noticed the patient had extensive stretch marks and a rather flaccid belly from multiple pregnancies. Afterward, I mentioned the patient's stretch marks to Vicky and asked if she had thought about where the patient's children might be. Vicky said she had asked the patient that question. There were three children. One of them had been taken by the state, one was in the custody of the maternal grandmother, and one was in the custody of the father.

This was an intriguing encounter. One of these women is twenty-nine, unmarried, well educated, gainfully employed, and childless. The other is twenty-six, unmarried, unemployed, drug-addicted, a prostitute, and the mother of three children who are being raised by other people. This begs a crucial question. From a biological perspective, which of these two women is better adapted to her environment? Or, to ask it another way, which of them will leave behind more surviving offspring, and have greater reproductive success? The answer, of course, is the drug-addicted prostitute.

Young people in the Western world today, if they are smart and responsible, can escape the burdens of child rearing. The example above compares two women, but the phenomenon is not limited to women. It is easier to demonstrate in women because parenthood is unambiguous in females. Several childless men work with me, and each of them has less reproductive success than the fathers of this patient's three children. Bright, talented, well-educated people are often less well adapted than their counterparts when measured in biological terms, such as reproductive success.

It would have been unimaginable to people a hundred years ago that a woman outside the confines of a convent would ever willingly choose not to bear children. Barren women were burned as witches or cast out of villages and towns. Even today, in the primitive places of the world, a barren woman is an evil thing, and her evil can infect other women. Such women are banished. Their bodies are buried in remote, unmarked graves. Fecundity was, and in some places still is, a woman's only value.

Western cultures have changed the perceptions of childless women, but the change occurred only recently. About fifty years ago, a paradigm shift occurred in the Western world, coinciding with the broadcast of *The Mary Tyler Moore Show*. This aired in the 1970s in the United States and became very popular among general viewers. However, it was initially highly controversial and almost did not air.

The focus groups who evaluated the show before airing did not approve of the concept and were offended by the morals of the main character, Mary Richards. She was a young, single woman pursuing a career in TV news broadcasting instead of pursuing a husband. She had no ambition to marry or to bear children and no inclination to live off the resources provided by a man. This was the first mainstream public woman allowed to lead the lifestyle previously monopolized by men. Only fifty years ago, the mindset of the United States underwent the paradigm shift to economic and personal freedom for women. Mary Richards did not earn her keep via reproductive services, yet the public embraced her character, although somewhat hesitantly. The *Mary Tyler Moore Show* marked a milestone in the social development of humanity.

Ironically, before taking on the role of the independently minded Mary Richards, Ms. Moore spent five years playing the role of the traditional housewife and mother, Laura Petri, in the *Dick van Dyke Show*. She transitioned from co-star status to having her own show. This was symbolic of the paradigm shift in society, as women emerged from their supportive roles in the patriarchal nuclear family structure.

People choose to limit or forego reproduction for many different reasons, some of which are admirable while others are perhaps not, but they are all valid. Some people prefer to devote their lives to other things: the betterment of the human condition, the development of a blue rose, the cure for cancer, saving the whales, or one of a million other causes. Others think too many people exist in the world already. Some simply feel they would be lousy parents, and they may well be correct. Others say they are too selfish to have children and would rather retire early and sample fine cuisines worldwide.

Some people have spent their childhoods raising ten younger siblings and feel they have already done their duty to humanity. Others would rather dote on their nieces and nephews at their leisure, then go back to their own peaceful homes and read a good book (or write one). Some people have genetic disorders, like sickle cell disease or Huntington's chorea, which they would rather not pass on to their children or future generations. For whatever reason, many people choose to suppress their reproductive instincts and surrender their places in the gene pool.

I once had a pleasant conversation with a young woman named Margaret, a waitress in a restaurant where I ate dinner with my wife and young children many years ago. Margaret was very adept at entertaining our kids. I asked her if she had children of her own, and she said she would never have any. She had helped raise her eight younger siblings, and she had had quite enough of child rearing. She had decided instead to go to college and become an attorney. Margaret represents that group of people who feel they have done enough to advance humanity by raising their siblings. They have no need, desire, or obligation to have children of their own. They are like the worker ants who invest in their siblings rather than their offspring. This option would not have been easily available to Margaret before about 1960.

Jane was a strikingly beautiful young woman in my high school class. A tall Scandinavian blonde with a flirtatious personality, she was always surrounded by hopeful young men. At our 30th class reunion, she was still beautiful. She had never married or had children. She enjoyed her good looks and her suitors too much. Jane chose not to have children simply because she was unwilling to give up her single and highly attractive lifestyle.

Ann and Dennis are childless by choice. Dennis has a hereditary disorder called epidermal dysplasia that causes unpleasant abnormalities of the skin, hair, and teeth. He does not want to transmit this disorder to children. Ann prefers to teach and study instead of raising kids. They married with the understanding they would not have children. They both have doctorate degrees in the biological sciences and are well-respected instructors and researchers at a university.

A young woman named Diane came into the ER one night with

lower abdominal pain. She was a pretty coed from the local college. Her roommate, another nice young lady, had come along for moral support. As I was interviewing her, I asked her all those questions one usually asks of a young woman with abdomen pain. When I asked her whether she might be pregnant, she responded, "No. I don't think so." Then she turned to her roommate and said, "Your dad has had a vasectomy, hasn't he?" The roommate assured her that he had.

Modern birth control has freed Diane to pursue her college education without sacrificing her sexuality. When she has the urge to have sex, she finds a convenient, safe partner in her roommate's father. As an older man, he is probably a more competent lover than men her age and is probably generous to her. Their sex is not complicated by any potential for long-term obligations and she has the complete approval of her roommate, an essential part of her social network.

Birth control and economic equality have liberated Vicky, Margaret, Jane, Ann, and Diane to lead active, full lives, including sexual relationships, without creating offspring. In the process, they forego the opportunity to propagate their genes. Of course, they are not alone. They all have sexual partners who also forego the opportunity to create offspring. Their genes are also lost from the gene pool.

It is not yet known whether a culture can survive when the best and brightest people opt out of reproduction. This option has only been available on a large scale for half a century. As a sexual strategy, it may be unsustainable. The loss of offspring must be countered by gains realized from the productivity of the people who have surrendered their chance to reproduce. Whether their contributions as scientists, teachers, attorneys, artists, and philosophers will offset the loss from the gene pool is not yet known.

<u>Idiocracy</u>

Released in 2006 without fanfare, this movie has acquired a cult following. It is a science-fiction comedy that follows the adventures of two thoroughly average people who are moved forward in time 500 years. They find themselves in a world where the population has been so dumbed-down by lop-sided breeding that humanity has become profoundly stupid. The two protagonists are brilliant by comparison, the smartest people in the world, and it falls to them to save humanity from certain disaster.

SEXUALITY IN THE WORKPLACE

In cultures that endorse sexual equality, men and women work side by side and have equal social standing. This generates a new set of problems by introducing sexuality into the workplace. When human males and females are near each other, their nature is to interact according to their genetic programming, i.e., sexually. However, there are laws that specifically prohibit any sexual behaviors in the workplace. Federal regulations forbid such things as touching above the elbow, referencing any body parts in conversations, and discussing sexuality or reproductive functions. It is not just socially unacceptable to compliment a woman on her figure, place a hand on her waist, or ask if she is pregnant. It is illegal. Off-color jokes and sexual chatter are no longer just in bad taste; they violate federal law. Such laws merely illustrate how difficult it is for people to suppress their sexual behaviors.

These workplace regulations are only marginally effective. Co-workers hug each other. Women talk about their pregnancies and labor experiences. Men complain about their wives and girlfriends. People share their health concerns and discuss their bodily ailments. They compare their Kama Sutra applications on their iPhones. They discuss intimate details of their relationships. Sexual chatter, innuendo, and off-color jokes are ubiquitous. Inter-office and workplace romances are common. On-the-job sex is one of the staples of office gossip.

Work is a large part of people's lives, in terms of the portion of the social network represented by co-workers and the amount of time spent in the workplace. Humans are not going to exclude sexuality from work sites. Too many opportunities and prospects would be missed. Popular magazines abound with articles advising readers on how to acquire the romantic interests of their co-workers.

Scouting for mates requires probing others to determine their interest and receptivity. The probing is visual, verbal, and tactile. Body language, flirtatious comments, and casual touching are all parts of the process. Such instinctive human behaviors will never be eliminated from places where people gather.

I overheard a conversation one morning at work in which an attractive female respiratory therapist was talking casually with three male nurses outside my office door. She was telling them, "I finally found a sports bra like we talked about. One with, you know, 'coverage' when it gets cold out." This pretty young woman had been having a running discussion with these three young men about the size of her nipples, the problems they cause when she exercises in cold weather, and her ongoing search for a bra that hides her nipple erections. It is tempting to discount this conversation as an innocent discussion of the technical design of undergarments, but there is no doubt this young woman's comments were titillating to the three young men, and she knew why she had their attention. They had zero interest in the technical design of bras. She was talking about her nipples, and they were listening intently. She was using her sexuality to get their attention.

Even in the absence of reproductive interests, sexual banter is rampant at work. Reproduction is an important part of life, and people talk about it. The highest incidence occurs in medical facilities and police stations, where no one is shocked by anything, and every facet of human behavior is fair game for casual conversation.

Nonetheless, casual conversations about sexual matters can be annoying to some people, and they get offended and complain. Such complaints must be acknowledged and acted upon. There must be some oversight and regulation of sexuality in the workplace. Mating behaviors in work environments must be suppressed, or nothing will ever get done. Sexuality is too distracting, and the actual work is usually much less interesting. Power differentials and privileged information give individuals unfair advantages over one another. Superiors at work have the power to make decisions affecting their subordinates' earnings. On the other hand, subordinates have access to information that can affect their superiors financially and socially. Workplace romances invariably generate conflicts and have negative effects on productivity, up to and including impeachment of U.S. presidents.

Unfortunately, the regulations regarding such behavior are often Draconian. They apply harsh penalties and classify suspected offenders as psychopaths and predators. For the most part, people want to engage in natural human behavior and interact with each other on some sexual level. As a result, the general population does not "buy-in" to the spirit of the regulations. Most people do not complain about sexual behavior among co-workers because they are not willing to be responsible for the harsh punishment.

Moreover, they do not want to call attention to their workplace. Complaints would lead to the strict application of the regulations to themselves and their other co-workers. This often angers co-workers. In the workplace and elsewhere, male-female relationships are rarely completely fraternal. Men and women continuously assess each other as potential sexual partners. They constantly monitor their surroundings for alternative mates. Wherever sexually mature human males and females come into social contact, this behavior will occur. Legislation cannot alter human nature.

DETHRONING THE STERILE CASTE

Recall Ann and Dennis, the couple who chose to teach and engage in biological research rather than raise a family. Richard Dawkins, author of *The Selfish Gene,* would say Ann and Dennis have chosen to concentrate on the perpetuation of their memes at the expense of the perpetuation of their genes. Just as prime numbers are the building blocks of arithmetic and genes are the building blocks of heredity, memes are the building blocks of cultures. Memes are the individual ideas, the distinct but intertwined concepts that make up a culture. Virginity at marriage is a meme. Each of the Ten Commandments is a meme. Einstein's famous formula, $E = mc^2$, is a meme. The idea that people should be governed by the consent of the governed is a meme. The concept of a meme is itself a meme, one created by Richard Dawkins.

People who write books, engage in research, or teach are propagating memes. People who proselytize or preach religion are also propagating memes. The non-sectarian teachers of scientific memes and the sectarian propagators of religious memes are historically in conflict. Over the past one hundred years, the number of people propagating memes in non-sectarian forums has increased exponentially. They have overrun the universities, schools, publishing houses, libraries, radio, television, and the Internet. They have smothered the churches, monasteries, and convents. The scientists, engineers, scholars, and philosophers now vastly outnumber the priests and proselytizers.

Throughout the early history of Europe, childless-by-choice was the privilege of the clergy. Religious institutions were the only storehouses of knowledge. Sacred texts were the only books. The Sabbath day was the only public education. Churches were the powerhouses for advancing philosophy, science, and art. Archimedes and his followers were sworn to celibacy. Nicolaus Copernicus, Galileo Galilei, Leonardo Da Vinci, Michelangelo, Raphael, Isaac Newton, Gregory Mendel, and most of the great minds of the Renaissance, were either clergy members or church employees. Many were homosexual priests, supported by a workforce of childless monks and nuns. They lived and studied in places devoid of the distractions and burdens of child rearing. They were the sterile caste. The reason religious institutions were able to maintain a workforce who could copy textbooks, plant gardens of peas, and sort the F1 and F2 generations by color, time the speed of pendulums, invent calculus, record the positions of the stars, and calculate the parabolic trajectories of cannonballs and the elliptical paths of planets is that ecclesiastical workers did not have children to raise.

Virtually all scientific advancements in the past two thousand years and up to about two hundred years ago occurred in religious institutions and under the supervision of religious leaders. With that knowledge came political and economic power.

Since the Industrial Revolution, a schism between the church and the universities has been growing. Over the last two centuries, first industry and then the government invested in science and research independently from the church. As they did so, they intruded upon the territory of religious institutions, which had previously enjoyed a monopoly on natural philosophy.

The first conflict emerged when science and the church diverged in the Renaissance. It persists today, and the political power between the two factions is balanced. The Roman Catholic Church convicted Galileo of heresy in 1632 for saying the Earth moved around the sun. Galileo's interpretations were shown to be correct before his death in 1664, but the Pope did not pardon him until 1992. In U.S. classrooms today, Intelligent Design has squared off against Evolution in a battle to be the dominant dogma of man's origin. As with the prosecution of Galileo, this is not a scientific debate about the relative merits of two theories. It is another skirmish in the ongoing war over a fundamental social question: Who will be in command of the collective human intellect?

Religious institutions are vying with public educational systems over controlling the reins of natural philosophy. Religion bases reality upon scripture, while science supports a version based on logic. More importantly – and this is the heart of the matter – religion provides moral guidance from a higher power, while science can only provide leadership based on human knowledge.

The same question is at the core of the great schism in the house of Islam. A war rages worldwide right now that began with the writings of Taqi ad-Din Ahmad ibn Taymiyyah (1263 – 1338). He rejected all innovation, calling it a cursed intrusion of Christianity upon the true religion. Taymiyyah was Sunni. He declared the laws of the universe written in the Koran were fixed and should not be further investigated. He rejected the Shiite branch of Islam and declared jihad upon Shiites because the Shiites accepted innovation and modernization of the laws by which men live. The Iranian Imams, the Taliban, and the Wahhabi are all followers of the writings of Taymiyyah, who, incidentally, was Osama bin Laden's hero and role model.

Until a few hundred years ago, it was obvious who controlled philosophy. Religious institutions had a monopoly on the workforce of childless adults. Churches owned the sterile caste. Religious entities controlled all science. Academics answered to the church. Churches and monasteries owned all libraries.

Today, birth control has relieved the lay public of their reproductive burdens. They have been freed to pursue knowledge without serving any religious institution. Lay persons are the students, postgraduates, researchers, and professors in public institutions around the world, plus scientists in public research facilities and government agencies, engineers and technicians employed in research and development in the private sector, application developers and information technology analysts, and physicians and learned professionals.

The number of people who pursue scientific and philosophical truth as a full-time profession has increased from a few thousand in the time of Galileo to tens of millions today, and virtually all of them are free from the ideological intrusions of religion. The astounding leap forward in scientific knowledge over the past half-century has been primarily due to the ready availability of birth control. This massive shift of human resources to the study of science has created a huge body of knowledge that threatens religion. The Free-Thinkers have seized control from the Faithful.

When knowledge supersedes religion, there are unintended, undesirable consequences. We humans have needs that religion fills. Gods persist in our scientific world for many reasons. Robert A. Hinde, in *Why Gods Persist*, explains this in detail. We need to know we are not alone. We need to understand the causes of adversity in our lives, find shelter in a parent figure, and ward off the fear of death. We need social structure, moral guidance, and a sense of purpose. Religion provides all this. Science is a poor substitute.

However, there is a greater concern when society openly challenges religion. The results may be disastrous when science goes too far and religion is driven back. The Soviet Union embraced the philosophy that religion is the opiate of the masses and tried to ban the churches. They failed miserably. The Soviet government could never get the people to buy into the idea of the state as an alternative to their gods. People need gods. No matter how grandiose their intentions, the intelligentsia cannot win the hearts of the masses. Anti-intellectual movements rise in revolt. Most humans cannot conceive of the reality intellectuals purvey. They can only assimilate the familiar narratives of religion.

The intelligentsia must be cautious. They must not push their agendas too hard. In *The God Delusion,* Richard Dawkins does just that. His arguments against religion may be sound, but his frontal attack is doomed to failure. Mere mortal humans need their gods. Man has a deeply rooted need for an omniscient and omnipresent parent. Humans fear an empty universe. Loneliness is a terrible demon. People get angry when non-sectarian knowledge challenges their gods. They commit religious genocide, slaughtering opposing groups. They take over airplanes and fly them into tall buildings. Mobs form and kill the intelligentsia. They burn the libraries. The dark ages return.

The Library of Alexandria in Egypt was burned repeatedly, once by pagan mobs, once by Muslim hoards, and again by Christian mobs. The Inquisition was undertaken solely to eradicate opposing scientific and religious ideologies. The Brown Shirts torched libraries and books in Germany in a prelude to burning the bodies of the murdered Jewish intelligentsia. As recently as August 25, 1992, two ancient, irreplaceable libraries in Sarajevo were shelled with incendiary bombs. They were intentionally burned to the ground in a religious war. (Incidentally, that was the year Galileo was pardoned.) People become unimaginably destructive when their gods are threatened.

Today, those most educated are the least likely to be religious, as was shown in a Pew Research Center study published on September 28, 2010. In a test of knowledge about the Christian religion, those who scored highest were the atheists and agnostics. This means that those least educated are the most faithful and the most threatened by intellectuals.

Only a week earlier, Pope Benedict spoke to the British parliament and advised that religion must not be allowed to become "marginalized" in the people's lives. He warned that "moral principles" rather than "nothing more solid than the social consensus" must govern public policy. Reason must not replace faith. Secular rationality cannot substitute for religious belief.

It does not matter who is technically right and who is wrong in the debate of science against faith. It only matters which philosophy best meets the needs of the people; which provides the best moral guidance. This is sound advice. It must be heeded by the social architects who would revise our cultures based on science. It is a lesson learned the hard way by the Soviets, Galileo, and countless librarians from Alexandria to Sarajevo.

Nowhere are moral principles more in collision with reason than on the abortion debate. It is obvious to some people that every human fetus is a person from the moment of conception, and interruption of that life is murder. It is equally obvious to people relying on social consensus (Roe vs. Wade) that a fetus does not become a human being until it reaches a certain stage of development, and until then, it is merely a parasite in a woman's body.

There is no middle ground and no way to resolve this moral/scientific conundrum. To be painfully accurate, half of the fetus is parasitic, derived from the father's genes, and half is from the mother's genes. She has been parasitized by a man. Remember, a woman cannot propagate her genes without propagating those of a man and visa-versa. Likewise, to be completely truthful, the two genetic portions of the fetus combine to form a unique human being at the moment of conception, and they are inseparable. That human being is destroyed by an abortion. This collision of truths is one of the many dilemmas upon which humanity now flounders.

Humans are generally more compliant with rules of a higher power than with regulations written by intellectuals. That is the strength of religion. The intelligentsia may be the driving force of a modern nation. They provide educators, engineers, political leaders, artists, and scientists who are the heart of advanced societies. However, the intelligentsia are mere humans. They have their faults and weaknesses. They are subject to criticism and disdain. The cultures that best utilize their great minds to serve the needs of the people will ultimately supersede all others. Over the past five thousand years, religions have been the clear winners in this competition. They held the reins of human intellect and brought us out of the Stone Age. Where we go from here, I do not know.

When humans developed large scale agriculture, it catapulted humanity out of the Stone Age by enabling development of specialized artisans and subsequent commerce of their goods. It freed people from the burdens of growing or gathering their own food and enabled technological advancement.

During my lifetime, humans have been freed from the burden of reproduction. This has enabled an explosive increase in the number of humans available to advance technology. A thousand years from now, if our culture survives, historians will identify this moment in time as a critical transition in human history. At this point, humans finally distinguished themselves from the animals by becoming so successful they could forego reproduction and turn their energies upon the arts and sciences. Modern birth control has enabled the great cultural advances of the past half-century.

It is beyond my ability to say where all this change in reproductive behaviors will lead. I can say we are currently witnessing the greatest revolution in human culture since the invention of agriculture. Much of the conflict we see in the news each day is simply the convulsions of a species in cultural upheaval caused by changes in our reproductive behaviors. Reproduction is the core of our existence. It is hardwired into our genetics. It cannot be easily cast aside. Any change in the rules of reproduction will have far-reaching consequences. Our reproductive strategies affect most human behavior, from a young woman's clothing choices for the day to major political decisions resulting in international warfare.

The door has now been opened to a new age for humanity. If we are to survive this transition, each of us must learn to live in harmony with our own emotions and sexuality. We need a better understanding of our genetic programming and a more realistic, comprehensive model of human reproductive behaviors.

CHAPTER THIRTEEN

MATHEMATICS OF SEXUAL DIVERSITY

The world is not divided into sheep and goats. Not all things are black nor all things white. It is a fundamental of taxonomy that nature rarely deals with discrete categories. Only the human mind invents categories and tries to force facts into separated pigeon-holes. The living world is a continuum in each and every one of its aspects. The sooner we learn this concerning sexual behavior the sooner we shall reach a sound understanding of the realities of sex.

— ALFRED KINSEY

Humans are highly versatile. They do not separate neatly into binary groups. The arbitrary assignment of individuals into categories such as male/female, masculine/feminine, or heterosexual/homosexual excludes those portions of the population who are the in-betweens and the others. Human sexuality is a physiologic issue – not a moral issue. Sexual diversity is just that – diversity – which arises from statistical variations in human anatomy, physiology, and psychology. As such, it adds to the overall adaptability of human beings. Like any other characteristic, sexual diversity would not be present unless it served some adaptive function. Humans would not be designed this way without a good reason.

Discussions of sexual diversity typically begin with homosexuality, so I will begin by showing that homosexuality is a statistical result of human sexual variability. It occurs simply by chance. More importantly, it persists in the human population because, contrary to common beliefs, homosexuals are effective reproducers. Most people who engage in homosexual behavior are bisexual and simply practice reproductive strategies that circumvent the standard heterosexual paradigm. Homosexual behaviors are common in animals other than humans and have existed in humans since prehistoric times. There is no logical basis for classifying such behaviors as unnatural.

Homosexuality is surprisingly common in humans and takes many different forms. To illustrate the point, here are some examples of people who have engaged in homosexual behavior at some time in their lives. These are either people I have known personally or people who are well known in the public eye. They are for the most part upstanding citizens with careers, homes, and families. They simply do not fit the standard heterosexual paradigm.

Karen is a tall, pretty, athletic brunette I have known for years. She was exclusively lesbian in high school. In college, she gradually assumed a bisexual lifestyle, which she continued into her professional life. She eventually married a successful attorney, becoming his younger second wife. She had two children with him before he died in an auto accident. She went on to marry another professional man and to have two children with him.

Karen illustrates the flexibility some people have. People can change their sexual orientation as they grow older. Karen also demonstrates the reproductive potential of women who are lesbians at some time in their lives. Here is a bisexual female who bore four children to two financially successful husbands. She and her lovely, happy family are seen in church every Sunday.

Sean was an elderly professional man when I met him. He was

still working well past retirement age, mostly because his skills were needed in the community. He was then a notorious homosexual, having been involved in several public scandals. His ex-wife was just as notorious for her bad temper and poor judgment. The two of them had three children together before she caught him in bed with a man and divorced him with a great deal of public drama.

This man was, at least publicly, heterosexual in early adulthood. That may be in part due to his age. He was young at a time when homosexuals were persecuted. After two decades of marriage and three children, his pair bond with his wife had thoroughly expired. She not only divorced him, but she responded with contempt and publicly humiliated him.

After their divorce, the publicity of his affair labeled him, and he adopted an exclusively homosexual lifestyle. This may have been a change related to his aging, or it may have simply been due to ostracism. Sean is not exclusively homosexual but bisexual, and he is an effective reproducer. He has children and grandchildren.

Brian worked as a receptionist in a local hospital for three decades and was a valued employee. He was well-liked by his patients, co-workers, and superiors. He never married and never shared anything about his private life with anyone. When he died suddenly of natural causes, one man in the community came forward and cried at his funeral, claiming to have been his lifelong lover.

Most homosexuals are solid members of the community. They just happen, by chance, to fall into the part of the bell curve that is across the centerline (to be explained later). Yet, they live out their lives privately and quietly, playing the game with the cards they were dealt. Most homosexuals and bisexuals are not marching in parades, cross-dressing in public, or calling attention to themselves. They are going about their lives, working at their jobs, paying their mortgages, and often raising their children, just like heterosexuals.

Devin came to me in the ER one night depressed and feeling suicidal. It was the age-old story of a lover's triangle. Devin's girlfriend was sleeping with Devin's best friend. In this case, though, Devin, the girlfriend, and the best friend were all female. Homosexuals fall in love and fall out of love in the same way heterosexuals do. They have the same temptations, the same betrayals, and the same drama and intrigue.

Late one evening, one of my nurses, Anne, told me the story of her first marriage. She was twenty-one, and David was two years older. The church was the center of their lives. They met there and continued to attend the church regularly while courting and after marriage. The courtship lasted a year, as did their marriage. Although they had no children, they seemed to have a perfect marriage.

Anne told me how she had come home one day to find her devoted husband sitting at the dining room table crying, with a bottle of whiskey, two glasses, and a tape recorder. Neither of them were drinkers, but he poured some whiskey for each and played the tape. The message was from him to her, explaining that he loved her dearly and thought the world of her. He had tried very hard to be what she, his family, and God wanted him to be, but he was gay. He was miserable, living a complete lie, and could not continue this way.

They annulled the marriage. He left their hometown and moved to a large city. Anne was devastated. She was left confused about men, sexuality, and relationships. She was very pretty and had no trouble attracting new partners, but she went through a series of troubled marriages.

This couple illustrates the influence of culture and family on an individual's perceived sexual role. These two lovers were following a classic script of Christian romance, which was completely wrong for them. He was acting out the part of a straight male and a loving husband, but it was just acting. She was acting out the part of a loving wife, completely ignoring any signs indicating a serious defect in their sex life.

Anne's husband exemplifies the conflict that bisexuals face.

There is no place for them. They are pressured to choose between homosexual and heterosexual lifestyles. This young man functioned in a heterosexual relationship for two years but remained miserable. He was genuinely concerned for Anne's feelings, and probably did love her, but his physical attraction to men was so strong that he was compelled to leave this very desirable woman and face disgrace in his church, community, and family. He ultimately abandoned his entire social network to seek a new life elsewhere.

Any discussion of homosexuality becomes mired in linguistics from the onset. Just deciding what constitutes a homosexual is problematic. Both males and females change their preferences over time due to internal and external influences. There is no conclusive data on how many people are homosexual, partly because the answer depends on time, place, and circumstances. If you count only those who identify themselves as homosexuals, about four percent of men and two percent of women are homosexual. If you count all those who have ever had a sexual encounter with a member of their own sex, the figures are ten percent and five percent, respectively. However, if you include everyone who has ever been aroused by the thought of a member of their sex, then the figure is as high as forty percent for both sexes. Humans are clearly elastic and versatile in their sexual behaviors.

Some animals on Earth are very restricted in their sexual behaviors. Most species can only have sex during a brief time of the month or the year. Most animals are constrained to sex with members of the opposite sex within their species. Most animals can only copulate in one position. Some animals are restricted to sex at one spot on Earth, with one particular member of the opposite sex of their species, and at one time of the year or only once in a lifetime. Humans are not like that.

Humans are extremely diverse in their sexuality. They can have sex in an overwhelming array of settings. They can have sex in any position with the opposite sex, the same sex, farm animals, vegetables, appliances, inanimate objects, and mechanical devices. They can have sex at any time of the month or year, and anywhere on Earth, in the sky, under water, or in outer space. Their individual preferences at any given moment are determined by their current libido levels, availability of partners, and a combination of genetic and cultural influences.

A PRIMER ON POPULATION DISTRIBUTION CURVES

Populations of living things do not divide neatly into two categories. Rather, they fall into poorly demarcated, often overlapping groups. They are distributed in bell curves. For example, human skin color is not simply black or white. Skin color varies over a continuous range. Most people fall in certain areas, but every point on the range has someone. Sexuality is that way, too. People are not just divided into male versus female, masculine versus feminine, or heterosexual versus homosexual. They vary continuously, with someone at every point on the range.

Dozens (if not hundreds) of genes control sexual behavior. Each of these genes has multiple alleles or variations. Maternal hormones influence their expressions during fetal development. Various social and cultural experiences influence sexuality during adolescence and adulthood. When so many independent factors affect a person's sexuality, individual sexual behavior becomes stochastic. In other words, it is randomized over a continuous range from extreme male behaviors to extreme female behaviors.

When random input from multiple independent sources determines traits, each source is like a coin toss. Imagine you have two coins, and you keep tossing them on the ground, noting the number of heads and tails after each toss. Half of the time, the coins will land with one head and one tail up. One-fourth of the time, they will both be tails, and one-fourth of the time, they will both be heads. The graph below represents this.

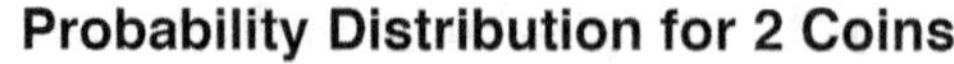

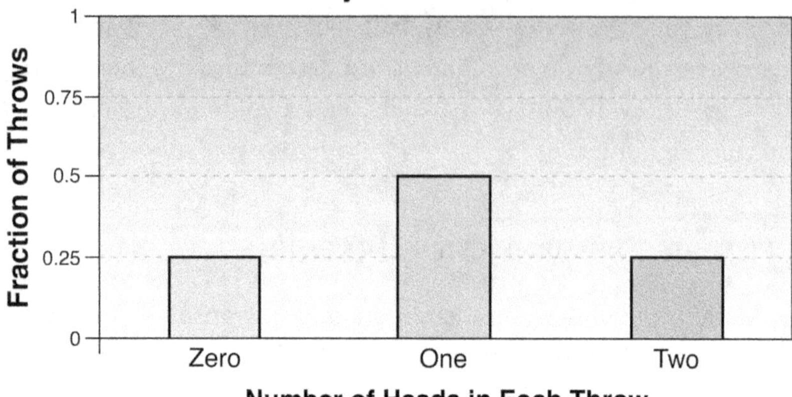

This result is the same as the distribution of color in peas discovered by the monk Mendel in his famous experiments with the genetics of garden peas. When a plant grown from a yellow pea seed was cross-pollinated with a plant grown from a green pea seed, one-fourth of the resulting peas were green, one-half were yellow-green, and one-fourth were yellow.

Now, consider the same operation with six coins. The number of heads will vary from zero to six with each toss, but, over time, the most common combination will be three heads and three tails. The next most common will be a two-four combination, followed by a one-five combination, etc. This is shown in the graph below. The row of bars starts to resemble a curve.

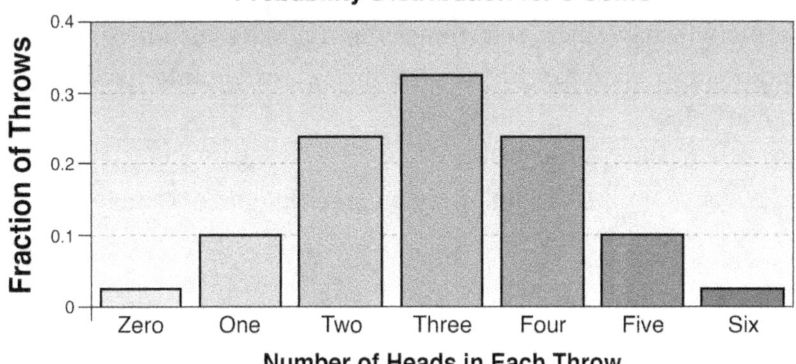

Next, instead of tossing the coins repeatedly, imagine you have a thousand people, each holding six coins. Each will toss six coins one time, and the number of heads up will represent some physical value. Think of the heads as genes that make people tall and let the coin toss determine the person's height above five feet. After all the people have thrown their coins, you will have a population distributed by height according to the following curve.

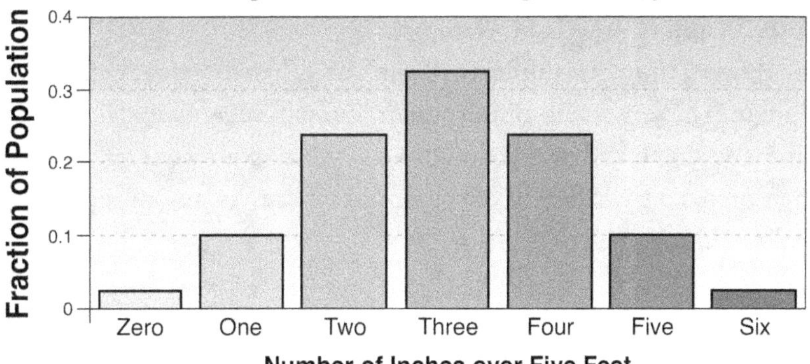

Of course, many more than six factors determine a person's height, and height distribution is much wider and smoother than shown in this curve. Repeat the experiment with more coins, perhaps twenty. The likelihood of a person having all twenty coins land on heads or tails becomes very low, but it will still happen. Most people will have their coin tosses distributed somewhere near the middle of the curve, with six to fifteen coins landing heads up, as shown below.

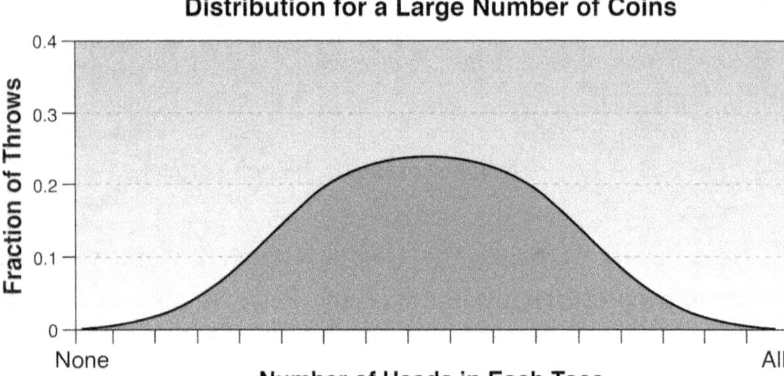

This is how biological populations are usually distributed. Characteristics determined by many independent factors fall under a bell-shaped curve, whether it is the length of antlers on male deer, the color of the fur on grizzly bears, the number of stripes on zebras, or the height of American women.

Height, though, is different from the other three characteristics. Humans have sexual dimorphism, which means males have a different shape and size than females. Women are generally shorter than men, so their height curve would be skewed to one side of the scale, as shown below.

Height Distribution of Adult Women

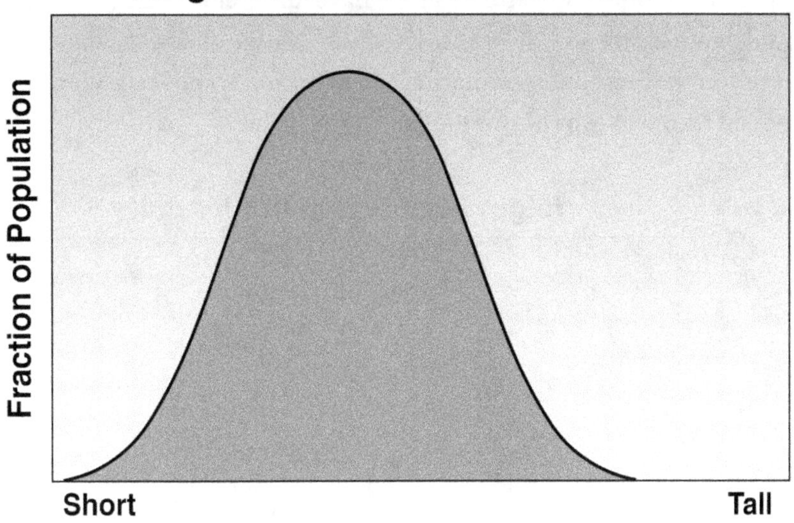

The height of men would be different from that of women. The men, on average, are taller, as shown below.

Height Distribution of Adult Men

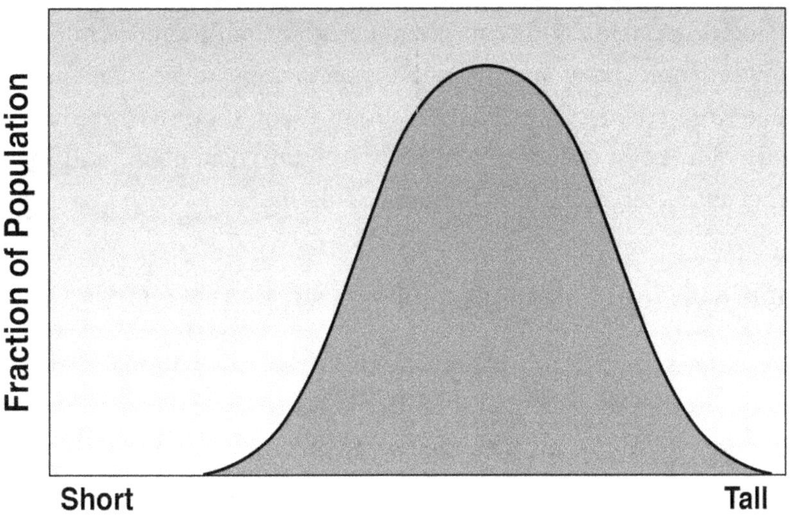

When the two curves are superimposed, a significant overlap is apparent. While men and women have different average heights, many women are well over into the men's range and vice versa. This is called a bimodal population distribution. The population is divided into two groups or modes.

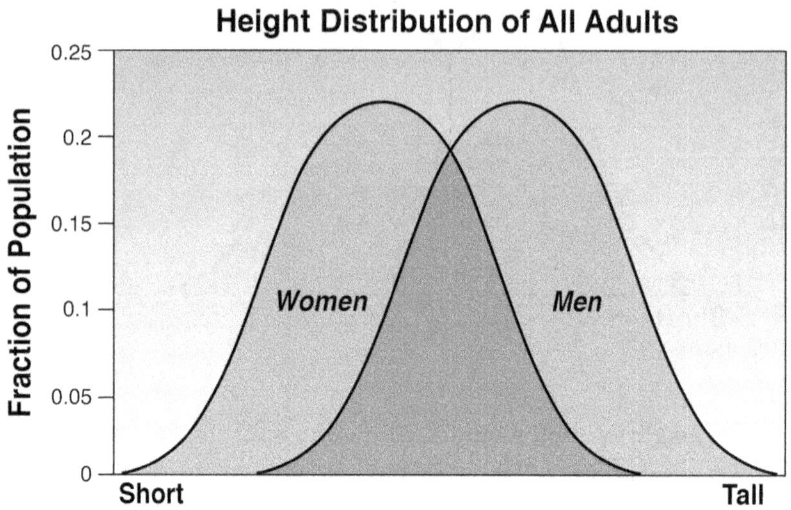

The same set of curves applies to many different parameters in biological systems. This case demonstrates the difference in height between men and women. Males are, on average, taller than females. This same set of curves could also represent shoe size, amount of body hair, body muscle mass, body weight, voice pitch, and many other characteristics of the human population.

POPULATION DISTRIBUTIONS AND SEXUAL DIVERSITY

Sexuality is a cluster of characteristics that have bimodal distributions. They are not divided into discrete categories. Women tend to be more feminine, and men tend to be more masculine, but there is significant overlap. Most women prefer sex with men, and most men prefer sex with women, but there is overlap. Women tend to fall in love with men, and men fall in love with women, but there is overlap. Some people are in the middle, and some cross over to the other side. The key to understanding human sexual diversity lies in understanding the effect of randomness on bimodal distributions of individual traits in a population.

Imagine a sexual-preference scale that ranges from heterosexual male behavior on one end to heterosexual female behavior on the other end. The right end of the scale represents attraction to the female body, and the left end represents attraction to the male body. The distribution of sexual preference in the male population can be represented by a bell curve on the right side of the behavior range. Most males would fall on the right side of the scale.

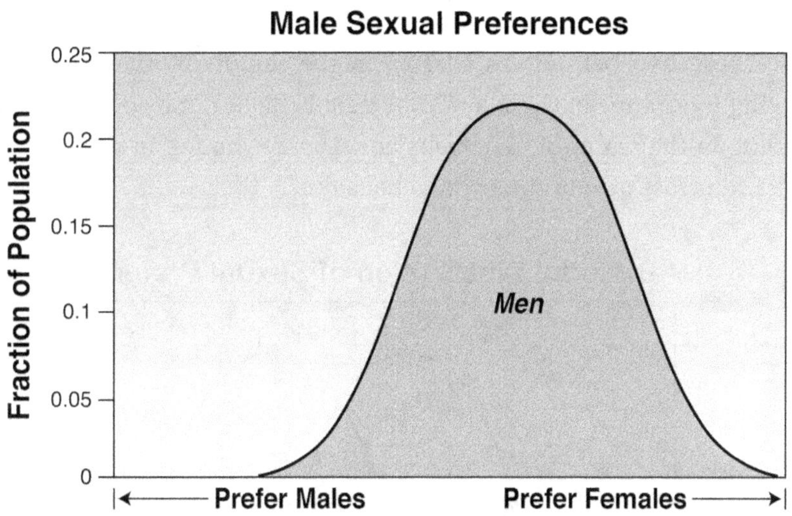

Female sexual preference can be represented by a bell curve in which most females fall on the left side of the behavior range.

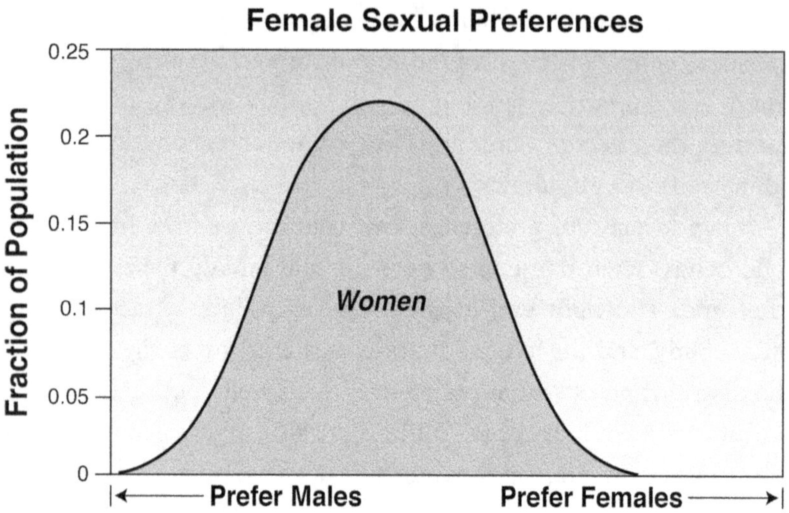

These two bell curves overlap in the middle, with some men falling by chance in the realm of female behavior and some women falling in the realm of male behavior. Those who fall in the overlap area can cross over in their sexual behavior.

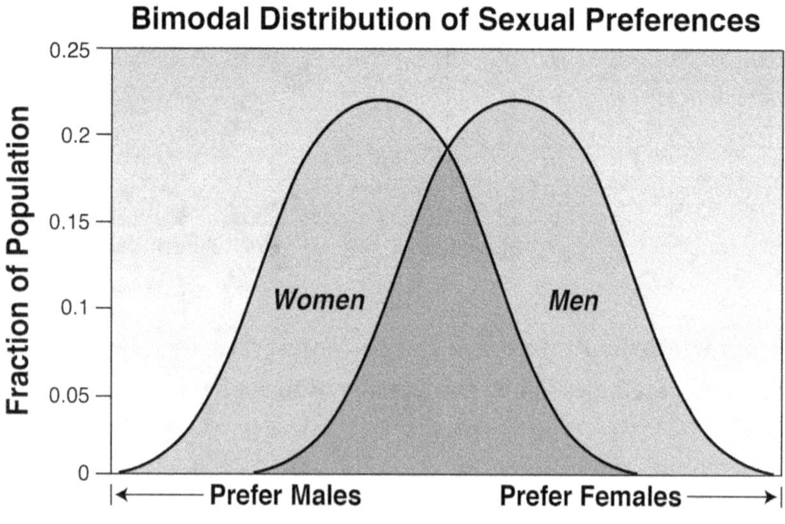

This means that for each sex, a small number of individuals will act strongly like the other sex in terms of their sexual preference. A larger number will have some ability to act like either sex, while the rest will act only like their own sex. These three groups are the obligate homosexuals, the bisexuals, and the obligate heterosexuals. Within each sex, the majority will be exclusively heterosexual.

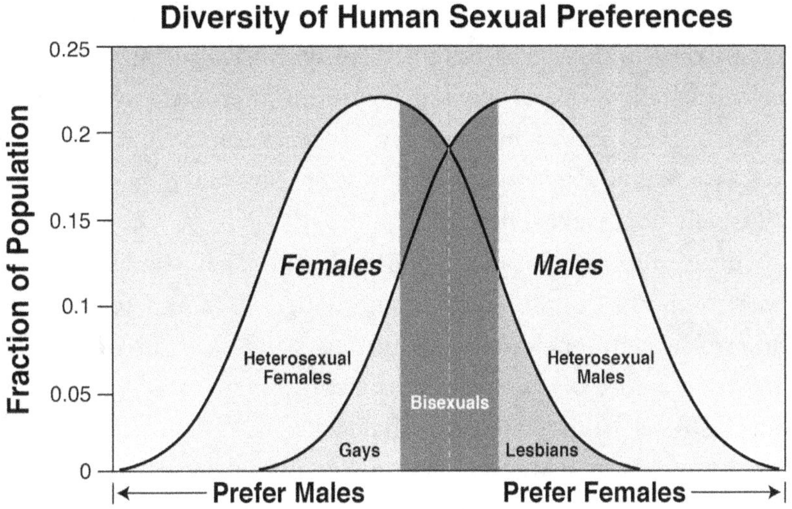

Many things affect the crossover behavior in the overlap groups. People are sometimes exposed to conditions where the opposite sex is unavailable. Some people live in cultures that condone or encourage homosexuality. Libido is variable, and increased libido causes people to be less selective about their partners. Under these conditions, members of a crossover population will use whatever partners are available. When released from constraints or compelled by loneliness, need, or lust, those people who are genetically able to do so will cross over to the behavior of the opposite sex.

For this reason, more homosexual behavior occurs in prisons or on naval ships at sea than in the general population. It is not because homosexuals are more prone to join navies or commit crimes but simply because many same-sex individuals are confined together, with no members of the opposite sex available. These conditions force individuals to choose between homosexual sex and no sex. Many people in the overlapping areas of the bell curves would choose heterosexual sex over homosexual sex if given the option but choose homosexuality over celibacy when the need arises. Under compelling conditions, some people can behave as either heterosexuals or homosexuals.

Most people in the overlap group are bisexual. Most women who, at some time in their lives, have had sex with a woman have also had sex with men. Bisexual women far outnumber exclusive lesbians. Likewise, most men who have had at least one sexual encounter with a man have also had sex with women. Bisexual men outnumber exclusively homosexual men.

This is one of the reasons it is pointless to label people as heterosexual or homosexual – they often change back and forth. Many homosexuals enter heterosexual marriages and have families early in adulthood before discovering or admitting their sexual preferences. Some lesbians accept short-term male lovers just to father their children. Many bisexual women choose women for lovers because men are too aggressive and dangerous. Many other bisexual women lead exclusively heterosexual lives to conform to cultural norms. Many homosexual men marry women and have families. They may give up their homosexual lifestyles entirely or have extramarital male lovers. Many homosexual men have occasional opportunistic sex with women. Some homosexual men are married to women only for the length of a pair bond and then resume their preferred lifestyles. Both men and women alternate back and forth between sexes in their pair bonds.

Likewise, it is pointless to discuss whether homosexual behavior is a choice versus a fixed trait. Obligate homosexuals, those on the periphery of the overlapping bell curves, do not have any choice in the matter. They simply cannot be heterosexual. Likewise, obligate heterosexuals do not have any choice. They cannot respond sexually to their own sex. They cannot engage in homosexual behavior. However, bisexuals do get to choose. For bisexuals, homosexuality is a choice, as is heterosexuality. My friend Chasity says, "I just love people."

At this point, the reader may be thinking, "So, who am I? Where am I on this curve?" Before addressing that issue, understand that sexual preference is not a dyad. It is not a question of whether a person is straight or gay. Rather, it is a matter of where one falls on the spectrum of sexual preference.

The graph represents sexual preference and is about physical arousal. Ask yourself what arouses you during sexual dreams or masturbation. Don't be distracted by the occasional hug or kiss in a dream. Those are just symbolic. Think about those dreams that include actual physical sexual arousal. Did they involve men, or women, or a mix? Gays get aroused in their dreams with same sex partners. Straights have sexual dreams with the opposite sex. A significant portion of the population have sexual dreams that include both sexes, and these are the people who can be aroused by the same or the opposite sex. They have the potential to be bisexual. Whether they choose to live that lifestyle is a different question.

Likewise, masturbation fantasies reveal sexual preferences. What scenarios do you summon to arouse yourself? Regardless of the public lifestyle you have chosen, you have a set of images and scenarios that stimulate you sexually. Preference is simply a question of which sex your physiology responds to. Is it male or female or both?

GAY GENES

The question inevitably arises whether people are born gay or born straight. Every person is born to be somewhere on the continuum from extreme male to extreme female preference. There is a place on the curve for every person where they are most comfortable. That location is determined by many different genes and by hormonal influences during development in the womb. Most of the population is in the obligate heterosexual area. A slightly smaller number of people are born to be in the overlapping portions of the bell curves and are bisexuals. A smaller number are in the periphery of the overlapping curves and are obligate homosexuals.

People can stray from their preferred place depending on their needs, libidos, and current situations. They can roam a certain distance when compelled to do so, remaining within a comfort zone. Those born to be near the center of the scale can respond to either sex when the opportunity or need arises. Obligate heterosexuals and obligate homosexuals are too far from the middle range to be that flexible.

Bisexuals just have twice as many chances for a date on Saturday night.

— WOODY ALLEN

The proportions of the population falling into these three groups cannot be accurately determined. Alfred Kinsey estimated that about forty percent of the population is bisexual. However, the number of individuals who exercise that option is not known.

The existence of a single gay gene, or even a small number of determinate genes, is unlikely. Sexual preference is not divided into distinct categories like the colors of Mendel's peas. Human sexual behavior is spread over a smooth curve in the pattern typical of multi-factorial stochastic natural systems. Hundreds of independent and random factors, including genes, determine sexual preference.

THE OTHER COMPONENTS OF SEXUALITY: SEXUAL ANATOMY, GENDER, GENDER PREFERENCE, AND LIBIDO

<u>Sexual anatomy</u> can be as confusing as sexual preference. People think of sex as a clear-cut matter of anatomy and genetics, so that a person is either male or female, but that is not correct. Some people fall into an overlapping area. Some males have a very small penis and

appear to be females. Some females have a very large clitoris and look like males. Some babies are born with ambiguous genitalia and cannot be classified anatomically. Rare individuals are born with both male and female genitals. Some people are anatomically female but genetically male because they have defective testosterone receptors. That is why genetic testing is required for some athletes.

Caster Semenya is a South African woman born in the early 1990s. By age eighteen, she had become a world-class runner. She is lean, muscular, and masculine in appearance, and she has a square jaw, a deep voice, and small breasts. She has never had a menstrual period. When she began to win competitions on the international scene, her sex was questioned. Testing revealed that she has no ovaries or uterus. She has a small, shallow vagina and two internal testes. She is, in fact, a genetic XY male who is insensitive to the testosterone produced by her testicles, so she has the external genitalia of a female.

Caroline Cossey had three X chromosomes and one Y (XXXY). She spent her childhood trying to be a boy without much success. As an adult, she underwent the hormonal and surgical transition to an anatomical female and went into entertainment. She was so successful that she appeared as one of the Bond girls in *For Your Eyes Only*.

In 1843, a resident of Salisbury, Connecticut, named Levi Suydam, was challenged regarding voting rights because he was suspected of being a female and, therefore, not allowed to cast a ballot. He was required to undergo a medical exam and was confirmed to have male genitalia. He was, however, also found to have a vagina from which, he admitted, he had regular menstrual bleeding. He was able to engage in vaginal sex with men, and he admitted to having sexual interests in women, but whether he ever had sex with a woman is unknown.

Anatomic sex in humans is distributed over a set of bimodal bell curves. There is a peak in the area of the average male genitalia and a peak in the area of the average female genitalia, but there are some individuals at every point along the entire range between the two peaks. The people in the valley between the two peaks must be identified by genetics. Even this can be problematic, though. Some people are not genetically male or female. Sex in humans is determined by the sex chromosome, which comes in two variants, X and Y. The human male has one X chromosome and one Y chromosome (XY), while the female has two X chromosomes (XX). Other combinations are also possible. Rarely, a child is born with two X chromosomes and a Y chromosome (XXY) or other combinations, such as (XYY), (XXXY), (X) alone, or an X and a fragment of a Y. Some people are composites, with two different genetic components to their bodies. Part of the body can be male, with XY sex chromosomes, and part female with XX chromosomes. Studies are underway to determine if this may be the cause of gender dysphoria. Some people simply cannot be classified genetically. Humans do not neatly separate into male and female categories.

<u>Gender</u> is different from sex. It is the sexual persona that develops as personality emerges during childhood, ranging from extremely masculine (think of Burt Reynolds) to extremely feminine (think of Marilyn Monroe). Some academics and scientists believe the brain comes in male and female versions. Others think gender is a learned characteristic. The truth is probably somewhere in between. Gender is like any other inherited, loosely defined characteristic. Each of us is born with a range of possibilities, and our environment determines the point within the range where each of us falls.

Most males have a masculine gender but to a variable degree. There are extremely masculine males, mildly masculine males, mildly feminine males, and very effeminate males. An occasional male feels so strongly feminine he insists he is a female in a male's body. Likewise, most females have feminine personas, but some display varying degrees of masculinity. Some females are only comfortable in feminine attire, dripping with estrogen and makeup.

Some are equally comfortable in pants or a skirt, in the workshop, kitchen, or nursery. A few women choose to dress and act entirely like men.

George Sand was born Aurora Dupin in France in 1804. After having two children, she left her husband and made a name for herself, figuratively and literally, as an authoress and a scandalous professional woman. She wore men's clothing whenever in public. She said they were more comfortable and less expensive than the elaborate women's costumes in early nineteenth century France. She smoked tobacco in public, preferring cigars. She publicly declared she did not need a husband, and she supported herself with her writing.

However, George Sand was not a lesbian. She had torrid affairs with powerful and influential men, including politicians, artists, poets, and musicians. Chopin was one of her better-known lovers, and she remained with him for years. She wrote profusely and documented all her affairs. There is only one hint of a romantic inclination toward a woman in all her letters and memoirs.

At the Pioneer Cemetery in Watsonville, California there is a historical marker over the grave of a remarkable person. It states, "Charley Darkey Parkhurst (1812–1879) Noted whip of the gold rush days drove stage over Mt. Madonna in early days of Valley. Last run San Juan to Santa Cruz. Death in cabin near the 7 mile house revealed 'one eyed Charley' to be a woman. First woman to vote in the U.S. November 3, 1868."

Born Charlotte Darkey Parkhurst in Vermont, she ran away from an orphanage at age 12 and adopted a male persona. Under the name Charlie, he learned to drive wagons and stagecoaches with up to six horses. He followed the gold rush to California, and became a legendary driver, known for his skill in handling a gun to fight off outlaws and highwaymen. He was also registered to vote. His secret was discovered only after his death, as friends were preparing his body for burial.

A patient named James was brought to our ER in cardiac arrest with CPR in progress. He was fifty years old, obese, and in poor physical condition, with diabetes and hypertension. Our resuscitation effort failed, and he was declared "dead on arrival." During resuscitation, all of his clothing was removed. An examination revealed bilateral mastectomy scars and female genitalia. Despite what his driver's license said, James was female.

The mystery deepened when his wife and stepdaughter appeared in the ER. James had been married to this woman for twelve years and had helped raise her now sixteen-year-old daughter. Neither the wife nor the daughter knew James was a female. The wife admitted they had never engaged in sex, but she explained her husband was impotent from his diabetes and hypertension. He had divulged this to her before they married. They slept in separate rooms and had never attempted sex. They had a Josephite marriage. The stepdaughter just knew James as her father. James was a woman who had felt so strongly about having a male gender she managed to convince all those around her, even her wife and stepdaughter, that she was a man.

A transvestite prostitute named Pandora was a regular in our ER for years. S/he was riddled with various diseases accumulated through his/her incredibly unhealthy lifestyle. We treated him/her for rectal fissures, prostatitis, urinary tract infections, perirectal abscesses, and finally for HIV and AIDS complications. Pandora insisted s/he was a woman, despite the presence of a penis and scrotum with testicles and the absence of a vagina. S/he did have well-developed breasts.

Pandora was once a loyal government worker in Washington, D.C. Under the name of Patrick, he completed his career and retired after twenty years in the Defense Department. He had saved his money and looked forward to the day when he could get a sex-change operation. He went through psychiatric preparation and hormonal therapy to change his body and develop his breasts.

However, Patrick was assaulted and severely beaten at a party one night and ended up in an ICU for months with multiple complications. He was eventually discharged but had been rendered penniless. Worse yet, he had become a poor surgical candidate due to the complications from his injuries. He could not undergo the surgical transformation from male to female. He lived out the rest of his life as Pandora, a tragic character stuck halfway between male and female. He had completely changed his gender but was unable to change his sex.

A wonderful illustration of gender can be seen in the movie *Miss Congeniality*. The main character, Gracie Hart, played by Sandra Bullock, is an FBI agent who utterly lacks femininity. She fights like a man. She does not wear makeup. She does not even own a hairbrush. In the movie, she is assigned to go undercover at a beauty pageant, playing the role of a contestant. This requires her to transition from masculine to feminine gender. Comparing the two genders in the same person is both humorous and instructive. It is important to note that her sex, sexual preference, and gender preference do not change in the movie. Her love interest in the film is a male. Only her gender changes.

<u>Gender preference</u> is the gender to which a person is attracted. This is different from sexual preference. Just because a woman is turned on by sex with a man does not mean she wants a masculine person to share her home. Most women like masculine men at least sometimes, but the degree is highly variable. Some women are put off by highly macho men, while others find the macho personality a turn-on. Many women vary in their preference according to the time of the month. They often find macho men fascinating during the two or three days near ovulation, and a bore the rest of the month.

My friend Elizabeth, a self-admitted lesbian, is in a long-term relationship with a woman. However, she confided she has a male lover she visits several times a year (about once a month if possible). Elizabeth is in love with a woman, but she prefers sex with a man when she is ovulating.

Gender preference in a woman depends, in part, on her hormone levels and mindset at the time. With a high estradiol level, a woman in estrus will prefer more masculine, strong-jawed, broad-shouldered men. At other times of the month, she will prefer more gracile, delicate features on a male. A woman may prefer a less macho male for her steady, long-term partner, but she may also seek a stud when ovulating.

Some women have a strict preference for feminine features and behaviors in their partners. These are women who prefer effeminate males or females for their pair bonds. Some women look for men smaller than themselves or want docile and subordinate men. Likewise, most men prefer to bond with women who have feminine personalities. Most men like domestic women who care for their appearance and want to nurture children.

Not all men share that preference. I knew a young man named Michael who lamented to me one day that he had lost several girlfriends over the years to other women, and he did not understand why. Michael has a gender preference for tomboys, that is, for women who have masculine personas. He encounters problems when he misidentifies lesbians as tomboys. Women who have a sexual preference for women are not necessarily masculine, but many lesbians adopt masculine personas to advertise their sexual preferences. They are trying to attract other women, but sometimes they attract Michael instead.

<u>Sexual preference</u> indicates the anatomic sex to which the libido responds. Regardless of a person's genetic sex, gender, or gender preference, the libido may only respond to a male body or a female body. A woman may prefer the company of a feminine personality, but that does not mean she can be aroused by a female body. Likewise, she may be inclined to pair bond with a macho male, but that does not mean she prefers sex with him.

Elizabeth is caught in this dilemma. She falls in love with

women, but she is not very satisfied by sex with women. She prefers to have sex with men because her libido responds better to male anatomy, even though her emotions respond better to feminine personalities.

Remember the bimodal bell curve distributions. Most male libidos respond to female bodies. Likewise, most female libidos respond to male bodies. However, the two populations overlap and contain people who have libidos that can respond to both males and females to some degree. Some people at the extreme ends of the crossover group can only respond to their own sex.

Libido is a curious thing. Some people simply have no interest in sex. None! Others think about nothing else and will take sex over food, family, law, and country. Nothing else matters! Most people fall in between, and for most people it changes constantly depending on mood, health, age, and hormone levels, environment, physical comfort, drugs, alcohol, medications, and abstinence. Libido is notoriously fickle. It can be turned on by a glance, gesture, or phrase, but even at the height of passion, it can be turned off, shut down, by a single word or gesture. Libido is under the control of internal factors and is also highly sensitive to external stimuli.

In a woman, libido follows a predictable cycle. It is low during menses and rises to a plateau after menses. It abruptly rises and peaks about a day before ovulation as the estradiol level rises. After ovulation, it recedes to the pre-ovulation plateau. About a week before menses, it gradually falls.

After menopause, female libido declines to a constant low level and women are unlikely to initiate sex without an ulterior motive. However, this loss of libido is offset by loss of fear of pregnancy, and by the experience older women have acquired in knowing what their bodies need. So, paradoxically, postmenopausal women may have less spontaneous interest in sex, and yet are able to enjoy sex more than they did in their reproductive years. This was noted by

Benjamin Franklin in a tongue-in-cheek essay on the wisdom of choosing an older woman for a mistress. (Franklin, 1745)

Superimposed upon this baseline pattern, libido in a woman – or perhaps I should say in a feminine persona – responds to gifts, kind gestures, and other evidence of devotion. However, it also responds to bravado and power at times of high estradiol. A safe environment and caressing, touching, kissing, and other foreplay predictably increase libido. Any negative feelings, such as emotional trauma, jealousy, fear, and physical discomfort, can turn off libido.

Males are more predictable than females, although they can sometimes be enigmatic. The typical heterosexual male libido responds to any woman interested in him. It can be a smile, a gesture, a few encouraging words, or simple intrusion into his personal space. Like women, men respond to caresses, touching, kissing, and cuddling.

However, males also respond to static signals, such as body shape and posture. This is why pornography has such a profound influence on males. They need nothing more than an hourglass outline in the 10:7:10 ratio to stimulate a response. Unlike females, who are selective about sex, males respond to all willing partners. A healthy young male is turned on by any female who entices him.

Despite that, human males are much more susceptible to internal influences compared to females. The male sexual response requires intact sympathetic and parasympathetic nervous systems and a healthy vascular system to achieve and maintain an erection. Many illnesses affect his critical systems, especially diabetes, cardio-vascular disease, and hypertension. Medications – especially psychi-atric and blood pressure – dampen the male sexual response, as does alcohol. Excessive use of illicit drugs, notably cocaine and meth-amphetamine, ruins male libido. The British navy used potassium nitrate, also known as saltpeter, to suppress libido in sailors at sea.

Emotional signals can also diminish libido. The male sexual response is notoriously fragile in the face of criticism from a sexual partner. Words or gestures easily bruise the male ego. Once it is injured and the erectile response is lost, it can be difficult to recover.

The male libido peaks in the late teens and early twenties and gradually declines. An eighteen-year-old man can have sex several times an hour. A forty-year-old man, when properly inspired, can have sex several times a day, and a seventy-year-old, under the right conditions, might manage once a week. Male libido quickly drops after an ejaculation, and then recovers over time. The time required depends on the man's age. In a seventeen-year-old, it happens in a few minutes. In a seventy-year old, it may take a week or more.

Libido is important in the overall theater of sexuality because it determines how much a person wants to engage in sexual behavior. It generates a great deal of conflict when husbands have high libido and their wives do not. It also is a major factor in determining whether a marginally bisexual individual will crossover to engage in an opportunistic homosexual (or heterosexual) relationship.

Unlike other determinants of sexuality, the libido distribution curve is not bimodal. It does not have separate peaks for males and females. The old belief that men have libido and women do not has been tossed into the trash bin of history. Both men and women are scattered all over the libido scale. Moreover, unlike the other distribution curves, libido is dynamic and not static. A person does not stay in one place on the range but moves constantly. When libido changes, it affects the expression of all the other characteristics. That is one of the reasons it is impossible to classify people as homosexual or heterosexual. As libido rises, people stray further from their set points. People who have been only heterosexual might stray into the bisexual range and engage in homosexual behaviors. Exclusively homosexual people might stray into the bisexual range and engage in heterosexual behaviors.

HOW THE PIECES MAKE THE WHOLE PERSON

Now that we have all these characteristics laid out on overlapping bell curves let us step back and see how they combine. It is important to understand that these characteristics sort independently. They do not necessarily mix the way one would expect. Anatomical sex, persona, gender preference, and sexual preference do not have to match. They do not come as sets. All combinations are possible, creating all kinds of unexpected diversity.

A few standard, well-recognized combinations encompass most of the population. Most men are masculine and prefer feminine women. Most women are feminine and prefer masculine men. These are referred to as *straight* people. Some masculine men prefer masculine women, that is, *tomboys*. Michael is one of these men, and he often occasionally hits on a mildly masculine lesbian, called a *boi*.

More masculine lesbians are called *butch*. Some masculine women prefer feminine women, the *butch-fem* combination. Some feminine women prefer feminine women, and they are called *lipstick lesbians*. Masculine or feminine men who are sexually attracted to men are called *gay*. A flamboyantly feminine gay man is called a *queen*. Some people "just love people" regardless of sex or orientation, and are called *pan*, short for pansexual. A person who has no interest in sex at all is called an *ace*, short for asexual.

Likewise, there are slang terms for heterosexuals with non-traditional preferences. An older woman who aggressively pursues sex with younger men is called a *cougar*. An older woman who remains attractive enough to be pursued by younger men is a *MILF*. A man who reverses the male-female role and trades sex to a woman in return for financial support is called a *gigolo*.

These are just a few distinct high points on a broad, multi-dimensional landscape of human sexual behavior. Human sexuality is not a simple two-dimensional spectrum like a rainbow. It is a complex sculpture containing every conceivable combination of sex, gender, gender preference, and sexual preference.

For instance, Thomas is an anatomic male who identifies as a female. He dresses in women's clothing and has a distinct preference for pink. However, he prefers sex with women. He identifies as a lipstick lesbian. He is in a long-term relationship with a woman who is pleased with the arrangement. I challenge the reader to name her sexual preference.

Likewise, how do we classify women who prefer men with Kleinfelter's syndrome? These men have one Y chromosome and two X chromosomes (XXY). They are typically overweight, soft-bodied, have lower muscle mass, and often have some degree of gynecomastia. About one man in a thousand has this condition. What is the sexual preference of the women who are attracted to these men?

HOMOSEXUAL REPRODUCTION

Homosexuality occurs in individual humans due to random chance, but that is not a complete explanation of homosexuality. We must also consider how the genes for homosexuality remain in the gene pool. That is to say, how do homosexuals reproduce? Obligate homosexual males do not reproduce, but bisexual males and homosexual females reproduce well. Obligate homosexual women are not aroused by men, but they can still engage in sex with men and are able to lead a heterosexual lifestyle. Females do not require arousal for coitus. However, obligate homosexual men cannot engage in sex with women. Male coitus requires arousal to maintain an erection. The propagation of genes for homosexuality relies upon bisexual males and homosexual females.

I will digress for a moment and discuss a disease called sickle cell anemia. This hereditary illness is caused by a defective hemoglobin gene. The normal gene is labeled Hemoglobin A, and the abnormal gene is Hemoglobin S. Every person has two copies of the Hemoglobin gene. Those with two A genes, denoted AA, are normal and healthy. Those with two S genes, denoted SS, are sickly, anemic, and in chronic pain. Without medical care, they die in childhood.

Patients with one copy of each gene, AS, go through life anemic and have occasional pain but survive and reproduce.

The sickle cell gene causes the body to make hemoglobin that crystallizes inside the red blood cells under low oxygen conditions. These crystals stretch the red cells' membranes and deform the cells into bizarre sickle shapes. The distorted, rigid sickle cells create logjams in the capillaries. This slows or stops blood flow to the extremities and organs, causing severe pain and tissue death.

The sickle cell gene is prevalent among the black population in Central Africa. This is curious. Why would a genetic abnormality persist in a population when it kills one fourth of the offspring before reaching reproductive age? Why does the gene not die out? For a deleterious gene to persist in a population, it must offer some advantage that offsets the harmful effects. In the case of sickle cell, the advantage involves susceptibility to malaria.

The malaria organism lives in the red blood cells and is carried from one person to another by mosquitoes. However, malaria organisms cannot survive in red blood cells that contain crystalized hemoglobin S. Patients with AS are resistant to malaria. In Central Africa, malaria is so prevalent that only persons with AS can survive to adulthood. Most people with normal hemoglobin AA die from malaria in childhood, and all those with SS die from Sickle Cell disease in childhood, but most of those with AS survive to have children.

Of course, *normal* and *abnormal* are relative terms. The AS combination is normal to Central African natives, and the AA and SS combinations are abnormal disease states that kill people. It is better to think in terms of whether characteristics are adaptive or non-adaptive in certain circumstances than to label them as normal or abnormal. Ultimately, the sickle cell gene survives in the population because persons with either SS or AA leave no offspring, while people with AS reproduce well and propagate both the A and the S genes.

Returning to the subject of sexuality, the lesson learned from sickle cell disease applies to male homosexual reproduction. Although obligate male homosexuals do not reproduce, many studies have shown that bisexuals reproduce better, reproduce earlier in life, and have more offspring compared to heterosexuals. The reproductive activity of bisexual males makes up for the loss of reproduction by obligate homosexuals. Bisexuals perpetuate the genes for homosexuality, and also those for heterosexuality.

Lesbian reproduction is not so enigmatic. Most women in the world today have little choice about when and with whom they have sex. Conservative religions and cultures do not offer women the opportunity to live independent of men. Lesbian women have the same reproductive obligations as heterosexual women.

A lesbian in Western culture can choose from a variety of ways to become pregnant. She can undergo artificial insemination, submit to isolated sexual intercourse with a male, or take up with a male in a heterosexual lifestyle until she becomes pregnant. A lesbian with a same sex partner has a stable platform for raising a family and constant access to a sexual partner without fear of unwanted pregnancy. She has complete control over when and by whom she becomes pregnant. When she does want to become pregnant, she can get higher quality genetic material than she could obtain if she were restricted to men who are willing to commit to a long-term relationship. She needs only to select a willing male and convince him to have sex with her, which is a simple thing to do when she requires nothing from him except his sperm. Most men are anxious to give them away.

The Genetics of Lesbian Motherhood

In modern Western culture, when a lesbian couple chooses to have a child, they often use sperm from an unrelated, and often unknown, donor. This avoids legal complications related to the parental rights of the donor, but it means that the child is genetically related only to the natural mother. Under primitive conditions, this would not have been the case.

Primitive people were highly promiscuous. They lived in groups of fifty to one hundred related individuals. The women had sex with many men in the community for many different reasons. They avoided having sex with closely related males, such as their brothers and sons. However, there was a high likelihood that a lesbian would be impregnated by a close relative of her partner. The child would then be genetically related to both female parents. A lesbian who is impregnated by her partner's brother bears a child who is the partner's niece or nephew. A lesbian impregnated by her partner's father bears a child who is her partner's half-brother or half-sister.

Sharing of relatives for sexual services is taboo in modern Western culture but occurred commonly in primitive cultures where siblings shared sexual favors with spouses. It still occurs in some extant indigenous societies. In some cultures, marriage consists of a group of siblings from one family wed to a group of siblings from another family. Under such conditions, lesbians would have had the same opportunity as heterosexual women to become pregnant and almost the same opportunity as heterosexual men to be genetic kin to their partner's offspring.

Of course, the male a lesbian selects should be unencumbered by a relationship with another female. Even the most liberal-minded woman may not take kindly to her husband impregnating another woman. Fortunately, most lesbians are close to a large community of men who are unencumbered by relationships with women. Lesbians can choose from the practicing homosexual male population. These men may prefer to live with other men, but most are able to have sex with women.

Helen was a healthcare worker and a well-respected professional. At fifty-one, she had never married. Early in her adulthood, she had wanted to have a child. She chose a man she liked and asked him to impregnate her. When I knew her, she had one grown son and three grandchildren. Helen owned a large home, which she shared with several women with whom she was sexually active. When the opportunity arose and the right man came along, she was sexually active with men. Helen illustrates the reproductive potential of a not-entirely heterosexual person. Although she prefers to live with women, she is a true bisexual, equally comfortable with male and female sexual partners. She is also a very feminine person and a talented belly dancer. For those readers who are curious, Helen chose a married man to father her child, but she asked his wife first.

Meredith Baxter, the actress, is another example of a lesbian with high reproductive success. After three marriages to highly successful men and birthing five children, she publicly proclaimed she is a lesbian. It would be more accurate to say she has now adopted a lesbian lifestyle. She is, in fact, bisexual. She has functioned effectively as a sexual partner to both men and women. Meredith has a feminine persona.

A co-worker of mine named Tina was exclusively heterosexual until her marriage failed, leaving her to care for two children. She was consoled by, and eventually fell in love with, a female friend who had no children. Once the two of them settled into life together with the children, Tina's ex-husband re-entered the scene. For many years, the three adults remained on good terms, co-parenting the children.

Meredith and Tina are good examples of people who are bisexual but live out a portion of their lives acting as if they are obligate heterosexuals. This may be where most bisexuals reside. Bisexuals outnumber obligate homosexuals but they are not as visible in the population. They lead conventional lives for the most part. They can simply adopt the standard paradigm of heterosexuality and fade into suburbia with everyone else. A Pew Research Center (Parker, 2015) study revealed that 84% of bisexuals are in committed relationships with members of the opposite sex. Only 28% of bisexuals have "come out" to friends and relatives, as opposed to 77% of gay men, and 71% of lesbians.

The other reason bisexuals are not visible is because public opinion pigeon-holes people into one of two categories, either heterosexual or homosexual. Once bisexual persons are known to be in a homosexual relationship, they become labeled publicly as homosexual instead of being recognized as bisexual. Such is the case with several of the practicing homosexuals presented in this text. Two bisexual women told me they have difficulty finding male lovers because they live with women in lesbian relationships. Men are confused by their enticements and are hesitant to respond.

Bisexual women have a special advantage in child rearing. A bisexual woman with children who finds herself single after a relationship with a male can subsequently choose a female rather than another male for her next mate. It is a less-complicated relationship. There is no risk of further pregnancies. Her children benefit from additional nurturing. The mother has a mate to help support her children without the mate being a danger.

A man has reproductive instincts that make him compete with a woman's prior mate. Even today, human males still occasionally reject, or even kill, the children of other males. The rate of childhood murder by stepfathers is ten times that of natural fathers. In my forty years of experience in the ER, I have seen only two cases of children murdered by natural fathers, but I have seen perhaps a dozen small children murdered by their mothers' boyfriends.

Like Tina, the great majority of lesbians who are raising children have retained the children from previous heterosexual relationships. In my research (unpublished), ninety-five percent of lesbian motherhoods result from an earlier episode of a heterosexual lifestyle. When a woman with children divorces and searches for a new mate for herself, she has the added burden of finding someone who will be tolerant of – and will not be a danger to – her children.

Tina and her ex-husband got along much better after she acquired a female lover. They may have felt more comfortable under those conditions than they would have if she were still alone or if she had taken up with a male lover. Because her new partner is female, her ex-husband is not intruding on another male's territory when he comes to visit.

Homosexual males are less likely than lesbians to be raising children, but it does occur. Usually, one of the males has retained custody of children from a previous traditional relationship.

The 2000 U.S. census recorded approximately 600,000 same-sex couples, twenty-two to fifty-five years of age, in the United States. Two-thirds of these couples were male, and one-third were female. Overall, thirty-nine percent were raising children below the age of eighteen. Males constituted forty percent of the child rearing couples, and females accounted for sixty percent. A quick calculation shows that twenty-four percent of male same-sex couples and seventy percent of female same-sex couples were raising children.

By comparison, sixty-eight percent of traditional heterosexual couples in the same age group were raising children. Lesbian couples have approximately the same parenting rate as heterosexual couples. This is enlightening. One of the lesbian mothers in my study sample told me, "Women embrace motherhood regardless of their sexual orientation."

Recall that females can copulate in the absence of libido. Under primitive conditions, lesbianism was simply not an impediment to child rearing because women in a promiscuous society had many reasons to have sex with men other than lust and desire. Lesbians got pregnant as often as other women. They did not need artificial insemination.

Homosexual males, however, did not have many offspring because males cannot engage in copulation in the absence of desire. The penis does not become erect. Unlike lesbians, these obligate homosexual males were spared the burden of child rearing. They were the Sterile Caste. Propagation of male homosexual genes relies on bisexuals.

Most research articles on excessive bisexual pregnancy have focused on gender-related harassment by peers as the cause, but this is speculative. The data only supports correlation, not causation.

Several other factors may cause bisexuals to start sex earlier and have more sex than heterosexuals. First, bisexuals are attracted to both sexes and have twice the temptation to engage in sex at an early age. Second, they have twice the opportunity, twice the number of potential partners. Third, adolescent sex is easier to obtain with a same-sex partner, as there is less adult supervision over the activities of same-sex friends. Bisexuals may begin with homosexual activity, gaining experience, and then expand to heterosexuality. Finally, sexual preferences are partly based on libido levels. People with higher libido are less discerning about their sexual partners and are more inclined to engage in bisexual behavior. By extension, bisexuals will, on average, have a higher libido than heterosexuals and homosexuals.

Regardless of the exact mechanism, bisexuals are more likely to become parents and become parents earlier in life than heterosexuals. Overall, bisexuals have a higher reproductive rate than heterosexuals. The losses from the gene pool due to absence of male homosexual reproduction are offset by excess fecundity among bisexuals, thus sustaining homosexual genes in the population.

Reproduction in a Sexually Diverse Population

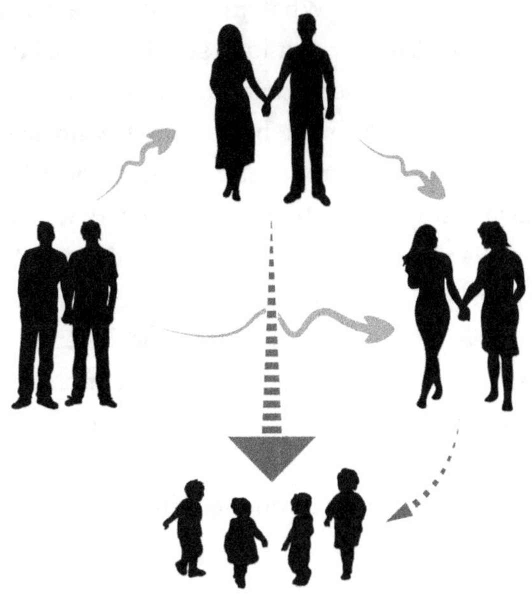

Most children are the offspring of heterosexual couples. Some, though, result from liaisons between: gay men and heterosexual women; gay men and gay women; or heterosexual men and gay women. These liaisons perpetuate the genes for homosexuality.

To summarize, sexual diversity is about much more than homosexuality. Humans range from obligate homosexuals to obligate heterosexuals, with someone at every point in between. But they also range from monogamous to polyamorous, and from asexual to sexually obsessed. Women range from frigid to highly libidinous on a monthly cycle. People range from completely cis-gendered to completely trans-gendered. Humans occur in every conceivable combination of sex, gender, sexual preference, gender preference, and libido. All this variability ensures a constant supply of people who can meet all the needs of a technical society. That is, after all, the whole point of walking upright.

Continuation of human society depends upon more than reproduction and child rearing. We are not just another mammal species with a unique set of genes. What makes us different from other mammals is that we also have a unique set of concepts that make up human culture. In order to perpetuate those, we need a wide variety of personal attributes. We must have people who are free to be scholars while others are reproducers. We need nest-builders who choose a mate and stay in one place and pioneers who take off into the wilderness. We need both men and women to range from masculine to feminine. We need hunters and gatherers, farmers and warriors, leaders and followers, socialites and loners, car salesmen and engineers, accountants and politicians. The richness of human culture depends upon a steady supply of dissimilar personalities. Ultimately, the greatest strength of the human species is its versatility. Sexual diversity is just one component in the overall adaptability of humans.

HOMOPHOBIA

...that they are endowed by their Creator with certain unalienable Rights, that among these are Life, Liberty and the Pursuit of Happiness.

— THOMAS JEFFERSON

Disapproval of homosexuality cannot justify invading the houses, hearts, and minds of citizens who choose to live their lives differently.

— HARRY A. BLACKMUN, U.S. SUPREME COURT
JUSTICE

Homophobia has multiple forms and causes. It cannot be addressed as a single subject. The conflicts between various sexual groups must be explored individually. Also, like many other human behaviors, homophobia is both an individual trait and a cultural heritage, and these have different origins. That is to say, the root cause of homophobia in a person may be different than the cause of homophobia in that person's culture. This distinction will be dealt with in greater detail later. The current analysis will only address homophobia in the context of the Abrahamic religions.

The most visible form of homophobia is heterosexual male ostracism of homosexual or effeminate males. It is primarily a learned behavior due to scripture references and peer pressure. Parents and the church teach boys that homosexuality is a sin, warning them about homosexual pedophiles and raising them to believe that all homosexual men are sexual predators. This is reinforced by enthusiastic news coverage of occasional pedophilia scandals involving prominent male homosexuals.

Fears are also reinforced when heterosexual males are "hit on" by homosexual peers, which is essentially the normal process that humans use to search for potential mates. It is composed of simple flirting, casual touching, and minor intrusion into personal space. It should be harmless, but it frightens heterosexual males in three ways. It reinforces their fear of homosexuals as predators. They fear their peers will identify them as homosexual and will ostracize them. Also, they fear they will respond and discover homosexual tendencies in themselves.

I doubt that any of these fears were present among primitive peoples when there was no distinction between heterosexuals and homosexuals. The Old Testament had not yet been written. Half of the indigenous cultures simply recognized that some people were not clearly male or female and placed those individuals in a group containing the "others" under various names. Those people were not ostracized or feared, and some were even revered. Children were not taught to fear them.

However, the other half of indigenous cultures were intolerant of male homosexuals, so there must be some root cause. I suspect the primary motive for straight males disliking gay males was economic. From the beginning of time, homosexual male couples have been wealthier than heterosexual couples simply because a male couple has two breadwinners and no dependent women or children. This creates an incentive to persecute homosexual males based on class envy. According to the 2019 American Community Survey, same-sex male couples have twenty-five percent greater annual income than opposite-sex couples, while only eight percent are supporting women and children.

Heterosexual masculine males also instinctively distrust effeminate males. To understand why, it is instructive to discuss a type of insect, a dung beetle. These are in the rhinoceros beetle family and display sexual dimorphism. The males of this family are much larger than the females and have prominent horns that they use for fighting over females and territories. Specifically, male dung beetles fight over piles of dung that attract large numbers of females. The male in control of a pile of dung gets to mate with the females it attracts. He will fight off any other male who approaches.

Some males in the species engage in gender mimicry. They are smaller and do not have horns. These males slip past the horned males unnoticed because they look and act like females. They browse among the females, waiting for the horned male to be distracted, mating with a female or fighting another male. They take that opportunity to mate with the females. This is called *sneaking* in beetles, but it would be called cuckoldry in humans.

Among humans, effeminate males integrate better with females than do heterosexual males. They have more feminine behavior and personalities and are more sensitive to the emotional needs of females. They have more common interests with females. Their thought processes and social skills are more attuned to female social settings. They are non-threatening, and because they fit in well with females, they will be close at hand when a female nears ovulation and seeks an opportunistic lover.

Effeminate behavior in males is a type of gender mimicry. It allows some men to have access to women through a different pathway than used by masculine males. I suspect this ability of effeminate males to cuckold is why heterosexual males have an instinctive distrust of effeminate males and try to drive them away. They don't like a man who is always hanging out with their women. Human males with effeminate behaviors are pursuing opportunities to reproduce. They are just using an alternative reproductive strategy. Masculine males are confused and frustrated by effeminate males who seem to be better liked by females for traits the masculine males cannot emulate. That is to say, the macho men get jealous.

Thus, male homophobia has two intrinsic causes. Homosexual males have an economic advantage over heterosexual males, causing class envy, and effeminate males have a sexual competitive advantage over masculine males, causing jealousy.

On a more general level, sexual preference is just one more attribute placing people in an identifiable group. All humans tend to sort others into the categories of "us" versus "them." The more a person looks or acts differently, the more they fall into the "them" category. Most homosexual women and bisexuals blend into society and go unnoticed, but homosexual males are much more noticeable. They are men living together without women, and they are generally wealthier than men with families. Some homosexuals stand out intentionally. They flaunt their homosexuality, and make themselves the focus of prejudice. This is why many heterosexuals who do not consider themselves homophobic are still offended by flaming gays and flamboyant pride parades.

The three Abrahamic religions, Judaism, Christianity, and Islam are notorious for their persecution of male homosexuals. All three base their prejudices on scriptural passages and the prohibition on non-procreative sex. However, there is scant reference to homosexuality in the Old Testament. The only marginally convincing passages are in Leviticus and the tale of Sodom and Gomorrah, and these are controversial. Many scholars believe they were altered or mistranslated for political reasons. The anti-homosexual slant reinforced the Israelite disdain for their political opponents, the Egyptians, Canaanites, Hittites, and, later, the Romans and Greeks, all of whom condoned homosexuality. Nonetheless, all three Abrahamic branches picked up the banner of homosexual persecution and carried it forward in time.

The only references to male homosexuality in the Quran relate to the story of Sodom and Gomorrah. There is an additional pertinent passage in which Allah states that all things are created in pairs, which is interpreted to mean there is no place for deviation from the strict male-female dyad. In the Muslim community, men should be men and women should be women. Men who behave like women are viewed with disgust.

There has long been a general condemnation in the Abrahamic religion for non-reproductive sex. This primarily addressed masturbation, but was also applied to homosexual sex, which is by nature recreational.

Jews, Muslims, and Protestants encourage their clergy to take wives. Their motivations for homosexual persecution are probably class envy, distrust of effeminate males, and simple prejudice. They justify it with scripture. Fears of having homosexual tendencies themselves amplify their prejudices.

The Catholic persecution of gays is more curious. We now know the great majority of the leadership of the Catholic Church is homosexual. According to Frederic Martel in his book *In the Closet of the Vatican*, eighty percent of Catholic priests are gay. Yet this organization of gay men forbids homosexuality among their congregation. They fight tooth-and-nail against same-sex marriage and equate Gay Pride with Fascism. This seems counterintuitive, but in fact it serves an important function for the church.

For two thousand years, the Catholic Church has been using homosexuality as a recruiting tool. Priests identify young men and women in their schools as possible homosexuals and confirm their inclinations in the confessionals. The combination of confessions and public condemnation of homosexuality steers gay youth into the convents, monasteries, and seminaries. While homosexual persecution is encouraged within the lay community, homosexuals are offered sanctuary in the church. This strategy has accumulated a huge population of child-free intellectuals and workers within the church organization.

Of course, church leaders did not intend to use homophobia as a recruiting tool. They were simply gathering more handsome young homosexual men and women into their social network for unrelated purposes, whether it was to offer salvation and sanctuary, or simply for selfish sexual reasons. They were not aware of the intellectual and political strength garnered by the church or the ultimate global impact. It was an unintended consequence.

This deception has now come back to haunt the Vatican in the form of scandals related to the very behavior they have publicly condemned and privately condoned for centuries. The Vatican is now fragmented by efforts to cope with the revelation of its hidden sexual culture. One conservative faction remains militantly anti-gay and denies homosexuality within the Vatican, maintaining the historical facade. These are the priests and cardinals who protected pedophiles rather than acknowledge homosexuality among the clergy. Another group admits that there are gay clergy, condemns them, and admits to the pedophilia problem.

The current leadership, under Pope Francis, acknowledges homosexuals among the clergy but adopts the strategy of "Who are we to judge?" so long as they respect their vows of celibacy. They have switched to a different argument, admitting there are gays in the church, but dismissing it as a non-problem because priests are celibate. In war, this would be called retreat and retrench.

A fourth faction openly accepts and embraces homosexuality in the church and the world. This group uses homosexuality as a weapon, bludgeoning political opponents in the Vatican by publicly outing them. As I write this passage, the Catholic Church is destabilizing. Ironically, worldwide acceptance of homosexuality may be the downfall of Catholicism.

Female homosexuality has barely been mentioned over the past two thousand years. Scholars have proposed many reasons, but I suspect the matter just remained "under the radar" of the men writing the rules. Men are generally unaware of the things women do while they are off with each other. Lesbians are not threatening anyone. They cannot cuckold heterosexual men. They occasionally take a woman away from a heterosexual man, but the man rarely fusses about it because of the stigma of losing a mate to a member of the opposite sex.

Lesbians do not attract as much attention as gay men. Heterosexual men find them intriguing because two aroused women are twice as interesting as one. Heterosexual women are neutral. Lesbians do not threaten the resources of straight women, and they might even provide a backup plan if needed. Homosexual female couples do not have any economic advantage over heterosexuals. They are generally at home raising their children. On average, their incomes are lower than those of heterosexual couples, so there is no incentive for class envy.

Lesbians are subject to some homophobia, but not to the extent of gay men. They may suffer the same simple prejudice as gays, depending on how much they stand out in a crowd. There are a few significant conflicts between lesbians and other groups. When a lonely or sexually aroused man approaches a lesbian and is rejected arbitrarily, he may become angry. Many lesbians have been subjected to "corrective" rape because they refused to accept men as sexual partners.

Some lesbians ostracize bisexual women for reasons similar to the ostracism of effeminate males by masculine males. Lesbians know how to compete against other women in their relationships, but they are confused when competing against men. A lesbian who dates a bisexual woman faces male competitors she cannot fully emulate. Lesbians also complain bisexual women are not real lesbians. They are just bi-curious, experimenting with alternatives and callously toying with the emotions of lesbians for their entertainment.

This again illustrates the difficulty of determining who is homosexual. The following is an exercise in Boolean logic that shows how difficult it is to classify people by sexual preference.

Boolean Logic and Homosexuality

Let the female population be divided into sets as follows (identical sets can be constructed for males):

Women who can fall into romantic love with women
Women who cannot fall into romantic love with women

Women who can be sexually aroused by women
Women who cannot be sexually aroused by women

Women who have had sex with women
Women who have not had sex with women

Women who can fall into romantic love with men
Women who cannot fall into romantic love with men

Women who can be sexually aroused by men
Women who cannot be sexually aroused by men

Women who have had sex with men
Women who have not had sex with men

Here are six pairs of mutually exclusive categories, which combine to create $2^6 = 64$ different groups of women. Women in any of the following groups might self-declare to be lesbians:

Any woman who can fall in love with another woman (32 groups):
Of the remaining 32, any woman who can be sexually aroused by women (16):
Of the remaining 16, any woman who has had sex with a woman (8):
And finally, of the remaining 8, any woman who is not sexually aroused by men (4).
Incredibly, women in 60 of these 64 groups could self-declare as lesbians.

Some lesbians are more exclusive, defining lesbians as only those persons who can fall in love with and be aroused by women but cannot fall in love with or be aroused by men, thus excluding bisexuals and asexuals. This definition requires a woman to meet four out of 6 categories. Because each category that must be met reduces the number of groups by one half, this reduces the number of groups meeting the definition of lesbianism to only 4 of the 60 self-declared lesbian groups. The other 56 are ostracized for not being "true" lesbians.

This exercise shows why it is so difficult to count the number of homosexuals (and heterosexuals) in a population. There is no consensus on what defines homosexuality. Statistics are based on self-declared homosexuals. Women (and men) refer to themselves as homosexual for many different reasons.

The past two decades have seen a staggering shift in the Western acceptance of homosexuals. Same-sex marriage, mostly illegal two decades ago, is now widely accepted. Homosexuality is no longer a matter of private shame but rather a topic of public discussion and a common plank on political platforms.

The widespread adoption of birth control and economic equality for women has crushed the paradigms of the male-female dyad and the nuclear family reproductive unit. People in the Western world no longer believe there is only one acceptable model for the human family. The rigid model of one man, the breadwinner, and one woman, the baby maker, is now gone. Western cultures now embrace a wide range of family models.

However, it should be noted that acceptance of homosexuality was not won by gay activism alone. The groundwork for social tolerance and equality in the overall theater of human sexuality was first laid down by Margaret Sanger and Mary Tyler Moore.

CHAPTER FOURTEEN
SEXUAL DIVERSITY IN THE NATURAL WORLD

Human homosexual practices have been labeled variously as "perverted," "unnatural," and "alternative," relegating them to the general class of "other than normal" behaviors. However, homosexuality is surprisingly widespread, and there is a wide variety of non-heterosexual reproductive strategies. We think of the sexual world as being divided into male and female, but there are at least five discrete sexes among animals, plus diverse asexual reproductive patterns and some patterns that fall in between sexual and asexual. Some scientists and doctors count five different sexes among humans, and others think anatomical sex is a continuous range from male to female.

Some animal groups, such as mammals, are generally divided into males and females for a lifetime. In others, the young adults are all male, and as they age, they turn into females. This includes many species of fish. Some fish species can change back and forth between male and female according to population demand. Other groups are true hermaphrodites with both male and female sex organs. All earthworms are in this group. Rotifers, some reptiles, and some birds have only one sex, which is called female by default because they produce eggs. What is "natural" in terms of sex is highly diverse.

Certain species of lizards, notably the whiptail lizards, have only females, and they manage to reproduce successfully. They mate using a rudimentary form of copulation. Two females court and then take turns mounting each other like heterosexual lizards. Although no genetic material is being transferred between the two females, mounting is still necessary. A female whiptail lizard will not produce eggs unless another female has mounted her.

In 1998, two male chinstrap penguins in the Central Park Zoo in Manhattan formed a pair bond lasting for years. During successive mating seasons, they engaged in the typical displays of physical affection that identify a bonded pair. They remained bonded year after year despite the availability of female penguins. One year a female penguin abandoned an egg, leaving it orphaned. The enterprising zoo staff gave it to the same-sex male pair, who then successfully raised the female chick to adulthood. We now know homosexuality is common among penguin species, and same-sex pair-bonding has been documented among 130 other species of birds.

Many mammal species that utilize polygamy as a reproductive strategy have several other characteristics in common. They are sexually dimorphic, with males being larger than females. Males mature later in life than females. Some males are not interested in mating with females but attempt to mate with other males. This is true among sheep, elk, gorillas, bonobos, and humans, to name a few examples.

Among our closest primate kin, the bonobos, homosexual behavior is rampant. All bonobo adults are bisexual. Same-sex relations are almost as frequent as heterosexual relations. Females have sex with other females, usually in the missionary position. They also engage in oral sex. Males have sex with other males in several positions and engage in a curious behavior called "penis fencing," the specific details of which will be left to the reader's imagination.

Finally, homosexual behavior has been present in human societies since the Stone Age. References to same-sex liaisons are found as far back as the earliest archeological records. In some Stone Age cultures, men and women were buried differently, facing opposite directions, and with different possessions or grave goods. Archeologists have found transsexual graves in which a member of one sex is buried in the position of the other sex and with grave goods typical of the other sex. Some men were buried as women, and some women were buried as men.

Behaviors of prehistoric humans are still observable, represented in the few Stone Age cultures remaining in isolated places on Earth. Ford and Beach, in their landmark text, *Patterns of Sexual Behavior*, reported that homosexuality was accepted by forty-nine of seventy-six primitive cultures studied, including eighteen American Indian tribes. Homosexuality is simply a part of the natural spectrum of human sexual behaviors. Like all the other primitive instincts in the human repertoire, it exists because it is a viable reproductive strategy.

CHAPTER FIFTEEN
THE STANDARD DOGMA

Most people I have known over the years were simply heterosexual. They took the straight path and adhered to the standard dogma. The women looked for men who could support them and protect them. The men looked for women who could give birth and raise their children. Both men and women looked for both long-term relationships and short-term relationships.

Men have been the primary providers with rare exceptions. Many women worked, but they usually earned less than their husbands. The men most often complained they were not getting enough affection (sex) from their wives, or their wives were spending too much money. The women most often complained their husbands wanted too much sex, gave too little emotional attention, or did not provide enough money.

Most people I have met still believe in monogamy, although many suspect something is not quite right with the idea. They hedge their bets with terms like serial monogamy. I think many of them recognize that the traditional dogma is seriously flawed. Their suspicions reflect dissatisfaction with their post-romantic relationships. Certainly, most of them are unhappy to some degree, and they do not know why. Usually, they blame each other or themselves. However, I have never heard any of them talk about pair-bonding. The linkage of pair-bonding to humans is a relatively new idea, one with the potential to alleviate the shame, guilt, and resentment that accumulates in long-term relationships.

Most people try to find long-term mates, and most of them eventually succeed. They do so with only a rudimentary understanding of the mechanisms involved in mate selection. They play their roles, follow their scripts, and make their decisions with no awareness of their effects on world politics or the course of human history.

For the most part, humans operate on their instincts and do not know why they do what they do. They just do what feels right. This was the case with my junior colleague Caroline. We can now answer the question I originally asked her. Why would she allow men to overrule the instructions written within her genetic program? The question must be broken into fragments, which can be answered individually. The easiest and most superficial answer is that her parents and religious leaders taught her to do so. They expended a great deal of effort teaching her that she should have only one sexual partner in her life and she should stay with him for her entire life. This would explain her behavior as an individual. However, it does not explain why she would feel compelled to continue the behavior. It does not explain what women have obtained from monogamy that reinforces and perpetuates the behavior.

Until a few decades ago, Caroline would have been compelled to stay with her husband because she had no good alternative. There was no other way for her to adequately provide for herself and her child except by attaching herself to a man and living off his earnings in exchange for her mothering of his children. What women obtained from monogamy was financial security. However, Caroline is highly skilled and employable, and she lives in a society that allows her to support herself. She can leave her husband, and she did.

Monogamy is not a natural behavior in humans. It is a human

invention. It was developed about five thousand years ago to accommodate the needs of patriarchal societies attempting to control property inheritance through control of paternity. It was redefined as a spiritual bond about a thousand years ago.

Monogamy persists because it provides the most stable family platform for rearing and educating children. Historically, it enabled the accumulation of a body of cultural knowledge, which eventually developed into technical knowledge. Those religions and nations that could keep the parents of children together long past their pair bond eventually became more technologically advanced than promiscuous societies. They could invest more in their children and educate them better. In the constant competition between groups of people, monogamous cultures surpassed the others economically, politically, and militarily. Caroline is a member of a monogamous culture.

Caroline frets about leaving her husband because she fears the effects of divorce on her child. She is aware that children do best in a two-parent home in our modern society. They perform better in school, have fewer behavioral problems, and are more likely to go to college and succeed in life.

Knowing all this does not make it any easier for Caroline to stay in a post-romantic relationship, and all romantic relationships eventually become post-romantic. Whether homosexual or heterosexual, couples fall in love and form pair bonds. After a few years, their pair bonds dissipate, their ego boundaries return, and this unexpected turn of events catches them off guard. Some couples struggle and eventually transition to a viable post-romantic relationship with varying degrees of emotional trauma. Others give up and resign from the failed relationship, never understanding the problems they faced. They leave one relationship and enter another, doomed to have the same outcome.

When a relationship between two people fails, the fault lies not in their morals or determination but in their failure to realize the pair bond is a term-limited process, and a transition to a different kind of relationship will have to occur after a few years. A better understanding of basic human nature and individual human needs will soften the effects of that transition. It will either improve couples' chances of a successful transition to a post-romantic relationship or reduce the emotional trauma of the transition to a post-marital relationship.

Of course, a life-long, post-romantic relationship may not be ideal for everyone, especially now that so many people remain childless. Recall the adaptive function of a post-romantic relationship. It facilitates the rearing of children through college. Childless couples do not have this social obligation, and they should be allowed to opt out of marriages without shame, guilt, or resentment. They have no obligation to each other beyond common courtesy. Like the post-graduate students, Dan and Alicia, they are free to go their separate ways. This also applies to most homosexual couples, and the absence of shared offspring is one of the reasons homosexual relationships are generally not as enduring as the standard heterosexual couples. By extension, couples who have raised their children should recognize that they have done their service to their offspring and society. Like my friend Katlyn, whose two sons had graduated from college, couples with grown children should rejoice in the successful completion of their marriage, cast off the social mandate of monogamy, and embrace their abilities to fall in love again with whomever they choose.

CHAPTER SIXTEEN
CONCLUSION

The initial question that inspired me to write this book was, "If humans were meant to live together as lifelong couples, then why is it so hard to do?" The answer is humans are *not* meant to live together as lifelong couples. Humans are not a monogamous species. They are a pair-bonding species. People choose to live together as lifelong couples because it solves a problem thrust upon them by human technological success. Humans have become so adept at using tools and manipulating symbols that the time required for children to learn all the basic skills of society now far exceeds the duration of the natural human pair bond.

Modern, highly technological cultures function better when humans live monogamous lifestyles. In the competition between societies, the surviving cultures and religions are those that encouraged monogamy and discouraged promiscuity. Monogamy is generally the best system for rearing children in our complex culture, but it requires that men and women live together as couples for a much longer time than is natural or comfortable.

Most of the misery accompanying a failed relationship arises from unrealistic expectations. Young lovers are disillusioned when their pair bond gradually expires. As their ego-boundaries return, they start to express themselves as individuals again. In doing so, they accumulate shame, guilt, and resentment, impeding transition to a healthy, resilient post-romantic relationship. This can be prevented if couples are educated about the true nature of romantic love. It is a time-limited bond in humans. Those who are aware that humans are not naturally monogamous can expect and prepare for a smooth transition to a post-romantic relationship.

Some pair bonds, even those that are irresistibly strong at first, are simply not destined to transition into stable post-romantic relationships. When the pair bond expires, couples may discover unpleasant things about themselves and their partners. They may find they have incompatible social networks. One of them may change sexual preferences or change life goals. Sometimes they just find they cannot stand one another, and they have "irreconcilable differences." These are natural outcomes when marriage choices are based on pair bonds. When this occurs, they should recognize that they got into this together, and they should help each other get out emotionally intact. They should continue to treat each other with courtesy and respect as they transition from a post-romantic relationship into a post-marital relationship (divorce).

A stable, functional post-romantic relationship is the best environment for raising children, but a stable, functional post-marital relationship runs a close second best. There are other good options: same-sex couples jointly raising their combined families, dioecious households, and matrilineal households. Ultimately, any family setting that provides a safe, loving environment, adequate financial support, consistent discipline, and wholesome values will produce healthy children.

Propagation is the goal of life. Some of us will propagate our genes, and others will propagate ideas. Our purpose is to carry genetic and/or cultural information forward to the next generation through the mixing of gametes and the nurturing of children. Ultimately, I must agree with Somerset Maugham. Falling in love is a trick played on us by nature to perpetuate the species. That is why fools fall in love.

Sexuality impacts everything around us. From a woman's clothing styles to the never-ending wars in the Middle East, it is all fallout from a design conflict between the pelvis and the kneecap. Recall the human female needs a wide pelvis to birth a baby with a large brain, but needs a narrow pelvis to prevent the knee cap from popping out of place when she stands upright. Mother Nature has provided human females with a compromise solution to this dilemma. They birth babies with small, immature brains.

Those helpless babies need a lot of care. They benefit if their mothers have a social support system. The social support comes primarily from hyper-sexual males, constantly willing to assist females in exchange for sex. Both males and females benefit from promiscuity. A hidden estrus ensures the females receive continuous support. Men have no way of knowing when women are fertile. In prehistoric times neither men nor women knew men had any role in making babies. The men were just in it for the sex.

Female homosexuality adds to the social support system for mothers. Male homosexuality and female menopause provide for intergenerational knowledge transfer. Bisexuality propagates the male homosexual genes in the population.

After humans learned about paternity, they developed systems to ensure proper patterns of inheritance. Men seized control of women's sexual choices by robbing them of their human rights. Religious dogma was the primary tool they used. Men replaced the prehistoric female gods with male gods who spouted moral guidance damning female liberty.

A wide range of religious dogmas sprang forth from the minds of men, generating conflict. Human males have always been inclined to fight and kill each other over access to females. Conflicting religious guidance regarding control of women just inspired men to fight and kill each other over women on a larger scale.

It can all be traced in reverse. Religious factions fight wars over conflicting dogma and a major part of that dogma is directed at restricting the sexual freedoms of women. Men restrict women's freedoms in order to control the paternity of children and ensure proper inheritance of wealth. They take this course because they cannot otherwise know the paternity of children due to human promiscuity and hidden female estrus. Those female characteristics are essential to the social support of mothers because human infants are so helpless. Human infants are born with immature brains because the size of the human pelvis is constrained by upright posture, which requires a narrow pelvis to prevent the knee cap from popping out of place.

QED

APPENDIX 1
"WHY" QUESTIONS

Forty years of work in the ER have taught me to ask questions carefully and specifically. The original title of this book was *Why Do Fools Fall in Love*. However, "*Why?*" is not a simple question. If you ask someone, "Why did you come to the ER tonight?" you risk getting answers like, "Because I had a ride tonight." or, "Because my girlfriend made me."

Of course, this linguistic hazard is not unique to medicine. Business leaders and project managers are coached on how to ask *why*. There is a wealth of literature on the subject, and the proper use is specific to the application.

When you ask why people engage in a behavior, you can get useless responses. Ask "Why did Romans wear shoes?" and you may get the response, "Because their mothers told them to." It is a correct answer, but not very helpful. To get a meaningful response, *why* questions about behaviors must be broken down into six different questions, divided into two categories.

On an individual level:

1. Why did the person first engage in the behavior? How was it acquired? Was it hardwired into his genes? Was it taught to him by his mother or his peers? Did he discover it accidentally?
2. Why does the person continue the behavior? What reward does he receive from it? What reinforces it? Does it feel good? Does it make money?
3. How does this behavior improve this person's survival such that he passes it on to more children?

On a cultural level:

1. How was this behavior introduced to the person's community? Did someone in their group invent it? Did they adopt it from another culture?
2. Why does the behavior persist in the community? What is the benefit received? How is it reinforced?
3. And finally, how does this behavior help this culture win out over other cultures? Why did this group of people displace cultures that did not practice the behavior?

As a simple example, <u>why do people wear shoes?</u>

On an individual level:

1. People begin wearing shoes when someone, probably a parent, teaches them to.
2. They continue because shoes keep their feet warm and protect them from harm. People with shoes can go places and do things that barefoot people cannot. They have access to more food.

3. People who wear shoes succeed better than people who have none. More of their children survive.

On a cultural level:

1. Some cultures started wearing shoes after a member of the group invented them. Other cultures then adopted the practice.
2. The behavior persists because it increases the community's health and productivity. Shoes are now required in most public places to prevent the spread of disease.
3. Cultures that wear shoes are more productive. They can tolerate more extreme environments, go more places, and accomplish more. They have greater economic and military success. Shoe-wearing cultures have replaced those that did not wear shoes.

In this example, a seemingly simple question has six different answers. All of them are true, but none can provide a stand-alone answer. When they are all combined, they explain why people wear shoes.

Next, let us consider a more enigmatic behavior. <u>Why do people smoke tobacco?</u>

On an individual level:

1. A person learns to smoke from peers or parents.
2. Tobacco smoke has both calming and stimulant effects, reducing anxiety and helping people concentrate. The act of taking a smoke break provides a few moments of distraction and relaxation. It feels good. Also, tobacco is

addictive and withdrawal causes anxiety, which is relieved by smoking.

3. Although smoking causes respiratory diseases in later life, it benefits younger people in reproductive years. People who smoke cigarettes perform repetitive tasks better. They are more tolerant of the tedious work essential to industry and parenting because they have periodic breaks from the work and they use a relaxing drug.

On a cultural level:

1. Tobacco was discovered by North American indigenous people who learned to smoke in pipes. Europeans adopted the behavior from them.
2. Tobacco became a major cash crop for the United States. The U.S. government actively encouraged tobacco production, commerce, and taxation.
3. The taxes earned from commerce in tobacco products provided funds for infrastructure and military projects. Supported in part by those funds, the colonies extended their domain across North America to the Pacific. The U.S. became the dominant political power on Earth, exporting tobacco worldwide.

Returning to human sexuality, consider the following questions: Why do people fall in love, and why do they fall out of love? Why do people in some cultures tolerate arranged marriages? Why were primitive humans promiscuous? Why do modern women strive to be (or appear to be) chaste? Why do people try to be monogamous? Why do good girls like bad boys? Why are some people homosexual? Why do some people fear homosexuals?

The answers are not evident in the setting of modern cultures but become intuitive when analyzed in the proper context. Each of these conundrums will be resolved by analyzing the behavior in terms of its initiation, reinforcement, and competitive advantage, first for an individual, and then for that person's cultural group.

<u>Why do humans fall in love?</u>

1. Individuals fall in love because their brains and hormones are designed in a way that causes their ego boundaries to collapse by flooding them with feel-good chemicals in the presence of their lovers.
2. They continue to be in love because it feels great while the pair-bond lasts. It feels wonderful to be that relaxed with another person.
3. Couples in love, working together to raise children, have more reproductive success than single parents. The two-parent division of labor provides more resources to the mother and child and gives the mother more time to nurture her children.
4. Our species inherited this ability from other creatures. This kind of one-on-one attachment has been part of animal behavior since before humanity. It is hardwired into our genetic code. (Or, if you prefer, God made us this way.)
5. Pair-bonding cultures benefit from dedicated parental rearing of infants and toddlers and communal rearing of older children. This frees mothers to continue reproducing and allows all members of a social group to provide general education to older children.
6. Proto-human cultures with individuals who could fall in love reproduced better than others because they provided better child rearing. They had more surviving offspring and displaced other proto-humans.

If parental pair-bonding benefits the children, why is the pair-bond time limited? <u>Why do people fall out of love?</u>

1. Human couples are naturally inclined to become intolerant of each other's idiosyncrasies after a few years. It is hardwired into their genes. Their ego boundaries return, and their infatuation ends.
2. They grow apart and separate to find new partners and form new pair bonds. It feels good to be free of conflict. They fall in love again with someone else, which is its own reward.
3. In primitive times, this reproductive strategy worked well. People enjoyed a succession of lovers in their lives. At any given time, most adults in the community were in loving relationships. They had more babies in each relationship.
4. Human cultures are composed of individuals who naturally fall out of love. Under primitive conditions, all human cultures relied on temporary reproductive relationships.
5. Falling out of love resulted in changing mates several times throughout a lifetime. This had two beneficial effects. It overcame barriers to reproduction caused by the occasional sterile mates and it increased social cohesion in the community.
6. The village or band raised children older than toddler age. All adults were surrounded by lovers and ex-lovers. All the children called each other brothers and sisters. All adults were mother and father, and all older adults were grandparents. When people lived in small groups, this reinforced kin altruism and social cohesion.

This reproductive strategy has now been mostly abandoned. Over the past 7000 years, societies that retained it have been overrun, destroyed, or enslaved by cultures that encourage nuclear families. This cultural change is the root cause of our relational conflicts. Our basic instincts have not changed in the past 7000 years. We are still emotionally inclined to find new mates when we tire of our current partners. But social obligations forbid us from doing so. One way to resolve this conflict is to completely abandon pair-bonding and just have loveless arranged marriages, which leads to the question, <u>why do people tolerate arranged marriages?</u>

1. Children in cultures that arrange marriages are taught by their elders that this is the proper way to obtain a lifelong mate. Relationships based on love are actively discouraged.
2. While devoid of love, these relationships are very resilient. Arranged marriages have low divorce rates, probably because the participants have no unrealistic expectations about their feelings toward one another. They do not experience the cycle of shame, guilt, and resentment that tears apart relationships based on love.
3. Arranged marriages are stable over the long term and provide sustained nurturing for children. They also incentivize men to invest in their children and accumulate wealth for their heirs. More of their children survive.
4. Many cultures independently developed arranged marriages. Other cultures adopted the strategy.
5. Arranged marriages provide solid nuclear families, with good control over children and inheritance. This stabilizes land and personal property holdings.
6. Assured inheritance incentivizes people to engage in commerce, improve their land, and accumulate wealth. Cultures that stabilize ownership across generations have more economic and military success compared to other cultures. They displace weaker societies.

Modern arranged marriages are, at least officially, sexually exclusive. The partners are forbidden from sexual relationships with anyone other than their spouse. However, primitive arranged marriages did not have such exclusions. Humans are naturally inclined to stray from their partners, and this inclination persists. <u>Why were primitive humans promiscuous?</u>

1. A person is promiscuous because that is his or her basic nature programmed in the genetic code. He or she is either told about sex or discovers it spontaneously. It begins as casual sex without pairing and extends to infidelity after pairing.
2. The person continues the behavior because it feels good. Sex is its own reward. Both men and women enjoy sex, and both benefit socially from sex outside their pair bonds.
3. A promiscuous woman had more than one man supporting her and her children. They would be more likely to survive. A promiscuous man simply had more children. Promiscuity avoids the risk of a woman being childless due to an infertile male partner. It improves reproductive success.
4. Humans as a species are promiscuous because they are genetically designed that way.
5. Promiscuity persisted in primitive cultures because it increased social bonding with members outside of pair-bonds and decreased violence between males fighting over females. Sex generates social cohesion in humans, just as it does with some of the great apes.
6. Promiscuity aids in reproduction in several ways. About ten percent of human males are infertile and cannot impregnate women. A promiscuous woman will get pregnant even when her mate is infertile. A pregnant woman with multiple

partners will have multiple men supporting her and will not be left alone if one of them dies or abandons her. Promiscuity enables sexual selection by women, resulting in prettier and healthier children. Those societies out-competed non-promiscuous societies (if there ever were any).

If humans are naturally promiscuous, and promiscuity has benefits, then <u>why do modern women strive to be (or at least appear to be) chaste?</u>

1. Modern girls are educated about the virtue of chastity from early childhood. They are taught to be ashamed of their bodies and their sexual desires, and warned of the dangers of boys, sex, pregnancy, and sexually transmitted diseases.
2. Women try to appear chaste to ward off ostracism and punishment.
3. Women who remain chaste, or maintain that image, have higher success in finding valuable mates. They obtain more resources for their children and have more stable homes. On the other hand, promiscuous women are ostracized, and adulterous women get stoned or beheaded or lose their husbands and alimony.
4. Men began suppressing female sexual liberties about 7000 years ago. They did so through religious dogma and civil law. Their purpose was to control paternity of children in order to ensure the legitimacy of heirs. In modern times, as population density increased, public health agencies have discouraged promiscuity to reduce the spread of sexually transmitted diseases.
5. Women in modern societies tolerate restrictions on their sexual freedoms in order to avoid harsh punishment from society. Men oppress women because they can be more

confident their legitimate children will inherit their wealth.

6. This succeeds as a cultural competitive strategy because men invest more in their biological children than in children of unknown paternity. They are more incentivized to accumulate wealth if they have legitimate heirs. In cultures that restrict women's sexual freedoms, the children receive more resources, education, and devotion. These cultures have greater success improving land, expanding commerce, building armies, conquering neighbors, and imposing their ideologies on other people.

Modern women strive to be, or at least pretend to be, chaste because men impose chastity on them. However, if women are only chaste under duress, and men are not chaste, <u>why do humans try to be monogamous?</u>

1. Modern children are taught from an early age that humans are by nature monogamous, and that the nuclear family is the only correct reproductive relationship. They learn this from fairy tales, romantic stories, religion, parents, and elders. They also learn that other types of relationships are shameful. They hear of girls "in trouble," of "failed" marriages, "broken" families, and "home-wreckers."

2. Monogamy stabilizes marriage by adding moral and religious obligations to a partnership. It imparts safety and stability to people's lives. It avoids the cost, effort, and danger of changing homes and mates.

3. Monogamy provides a stable social environment for raising children to adulthood in our modern, complex society. Children from two-parent homes have a higher survival rate and more economic success. (Note that until

the appearance of birth control, these affluent offspring had more surviving children of their own. However, that is not true today. In an alarming trend, affluent couples are now having fewer children.)

4. Religious and political leaders created the concept of monogamy about a thousand years ago to stabilize land holdings and aristocratic titles. (Note this is different from the fidelity imposed on females by males 7000 years ago).

5. Monogamy persists in society because it stabilizes marriages and property ownership, decreases paternal uncertainty, and motivates fathers to invest in their children, creating more productive members of society.

6. Monogamous cultures with nuclear families raise and educate their children continuously into adulthood. Fathers invest in their children and accumulate wealth for the benefit of their heirs. They produce young adults who are more educated, wealthy, creative, and able to make the most of their opportunities in life. They out-compete other cultures.

The nuclear family makes good sense, but humans are not that rational. They are driven more by emotions and hormones than logic. In the process of finding mates, both men and women do some very foolish things. To illustrate, let us ask, <u>why do good girls like bad boys?</u>

1. Women are naturally attracted to men who have enough excess energy and intelligence to do dangerous things and get away with it. It is part of the female design. Women are attracted to bravado.

2. Such men are generally less restricted in their behaviors. They are more spontaneous, creative, inventive, and

entertaining. Women like being with them because they are simply more fun.

3. Males who have the talent to misbehave without consequences tend to be more intelligent and socially successful compared to their cohorts. They acquire more political power and wealth. The women who mate with them get a higher quality of genes for their offspring. They have higher survival rates.

4. This is a natural characteristic of human females and many other female vertebrates. It is hard-wired into their genetics. It is a legitimate device for selecting a male with high genetic value. It was widely exploited back when women had sexual freedom.

5. Today, when women throw themselves at disreputable men or those men take advantage of women, it is often considered scandalous. Yet the behavior persists, whether in rock band groupies or White House interns. In the remote past though, there was no reason for condemnation. Both men and women were happy and comfortable with the system. The women's husbands did not complain because promiscuity was the rule, and they did not understand the role of sex in creating babies. They did not know they were being cuckolded. Cultures that allowed women to enjoy sexual freedom had smarter, healthier, and prettier children and happier men and women.

6. Ancient human societies that allowed sexual selection by women had more children with physical strength, intelligence, and creativity. It improved the gene pool. They were able to build stronger militaries and overrun other cultures. After women lost their sexual freedoms, newer cultures emphasized extended paternal investments in children, displacing the old cultures.

However, that did not change the basic nature of human females. Good girls still like bad boys.

Let us now explore why some women prefer other women over men. <u>Why are some women homosexual?</u>

1. Some women are homosexual because that is where they fall on the population distribution bell curve. Or, if you prefer, that is how God made them. They engage in homosexual behavior because they have the ability. They discover it in themselves or learn about it from peers.
2. They continue the behavior because they get the same pleasure from women that other women get from men. Many researchers (and many lesbians) claim they get better sex than straight women.
3. They do have sex with men, just not as often and not for the same reasons as heterosexual women. They get pregnant, and they raise their children well. They are generally not as financially secure as heterosexual women, but their children get more nurturing by having two mothers.
4. Female homosexuality has been in the primate line since before there were humans. We inherited it from them, or, alternatively, God used some of the primate sub-systems when designing humans.
5. Female homosexual culture persists because it works well for rearing children. Lesbians have some advantages over heterosexual women. For example, their children are not exposed to danger from an unrelated adult male in the home.
6. Cultures that allow female couples to raise families have some advantages over those that do not. For instance, when war causes many men to die, these women have the option of bonding with other women as an

alternative. These cultures have higher offspring survival, displacing other societies.

On the individual level, the reasons underlying male homosexuality are similar to those for females, but they differ on the cultural level. <u>Why are some men homosexual?</u>

1. Some men are homosexual because that is where they fall on the population distribution bell curve. Or, if you prefer, that is how God made them. In any case, they engage in homosexual behavior because they can. They discover it in themselves or learn about it from peers.
2. They continue the behavior because they get the same pleasure from men that other men get from women. Sex is its own reward.
3. Although obligate homosexual men do not have offspring, bisexual men have more children than heterosexual men. In that way, homosexual genes are propagated to the next generation.
4. Male homosexuality has been in the primate line since before humanity existed. People inherited it from them, or, if you prefer, God used some of the primate subsystems when designing humans.
5. Cultures condoning male homosexuality benefit from a sterile caste. These are persons who are not burdened by the duties of child-rearing and have the free time to serve as repositories of knowledge in the community. They are the holy men, observers, teachers, philosophers, scholars, and academics.
6. Cultures that tolerate homosexual males are more able to accumulate knowledge from one generation to the next, creating science, government, art, music, and advanced societies. Also, homosexual males do not fight over women. They are less likely to murder other men in the

community. This leaves more males available for the defense and provision of the group. Male homosexuals increase the survival of a tribe or culture, which then out-competes other tribes or cultures.

If homosexuality benefits the community, why is it condemned? Opinions vary widely among cultures and religions. Many cultures accept a wide range of sexual diversity as normal human behavior. In some societies, both ancient and modern, homosexuals were revered, and yet some cultures ostracize homosexuals. Questions regarding homophobia must be asked in the context of a particular religion or culture. <u>Why are Christian men homophobic?</u>

1. Male Christian children are taught to fear gay males as pedophiles. Adult heterosexual men have motives to dislike gay men, including class envy, jealousy, and simple prejudice.
2. These prejudices are reinforced by casual contact with homosexual peers, by peer pressure from heterosexuals, and by media attention to pedophilia perpetrated by prominent homosexual men.
3. Heterosexual parents have more offspring than homosexual males, and pass their fears and prejudices on to their children.
4. Cultural condemnation of homosexuals first arose among the Israelites and was a politically motivated rejection of the local Canaanite, Greek, and Roman cultures. It was later adopted by Christians, based on Old Testament scripture. Scriptures were used to reinforce the intrinsic motives for homophobia.
5. Historically, homophobia served Christianity well. It concentrated the non-child rearing population within the church, creating a monopoly on intellectuals and childless workers. Monastic scholars went on to develop

math, science, philosophy, art, and music, building upon and surpassing Greek, Roman, and Arab achievements. Christian cultures benefited economically.

6. Scientific knowledge blossomed in the monasteries, libraries, and universities. This led to better ships, weaponry, and logistics. Christian armies drove the Muslims out of Europe. Christians colonized Africa and enslaved much of its population. Christian civilization spread across the Atlantic and displaced the pagan indigenous cultures of the New World. The Christian population rapidly expanded and became the dominant religion on Earth, spreading homophobia and their unique recruiting tactics all over the world.

It is interesting to note that the New World was overrun by Christian culture, rather than Muslim, Jewish, Buddhist, Sikh, or Hindu. Some of these groups, such as Buddhists, are not aggressive by nature, but others, particularly the Muslims, are extremely expansionist. Yet Christians took unopposed possession of North and South America. This occurred because Christian culture was militarily and economically superior to other religions, due to the Catholic accumulation of homosexual scholars and academics. The financial and political success of Christianity is not due to its ideology, but rather to its peculiar policies regarding homosexuality.

There are many more questions about human behavior that would benefit from this type of analysis. For those who are up to the challenge, I would suggest starting with something easy, such as: Why do people drink alcohol? A much greater challenge would be: Why do people watch professional sports? (Hint: For sports, the answers are different for men and women spectators, and for men's and women's sports.)

APPENDIX 2
SEXUALITY AS REVEALED IN HUMOR

Humor is a powerful teaching tool. Jokes keep the readers' interest. They also open a special window into the workings of the mind, revealing truths. A joke cannot be funny unless it is based on a plausible premise. It is often the conflict between different truths or different versions of reality that is funny. Laughter is how humans deal with that conflict. Consider the following conversation between two teenagers, adapted from a Zits comic strip.

Boy says to girl, "Do you like Guinea pigs?"
She responds, "Oh! I love Guinea pigs."
He says, "Wonderful! So do I. Let's get together and compare recipes."

The sudden, unexpected reversal of the boy's intentions creates a conflict, which some people will interpret as pathos or cruelty and others will find funny. This sort of humor illustrates the relationship between comedy and tragedy that often confuses beginning students of literature. Humor is a mechanism humans use to deal with conflict. Laughter reduces stress.

This joke reveals a profound truth. The word *love* can mean many different things, and not all of them are beneficial to the object of that love. The girl uses *love* to mean affection, while the boy uses it to talk about food. The conflict between the two nearly opposite meanings of *love* is interpreted as humorous.

The joke only works because the two opposing realities exist. On the one hand, people adore Guinea pigs and keep them as pets. On the other hand, Guinea pigs were originally grown for food, and still are in South America. The sudden intrusion of the latter reality upon the girl and her adored pet is interpreted as humorous. The joke simply would not work if inedible objects like hand tools or Ming Dynasty vases were substituted for the Guinea pigs. The premise has to be plausible in order for the joke to be funny.

Many sources of information about relationships can deceive, but jokes are constrained to the truth. Off-color jokes provide a delightfully honest insight into the workings of human reproductive relationships. Every good joke contains a lesson to be learned.

When a thing is funny, search it for a hidden truth.

— GEORGE BERNARD SHAW

Humor is the affectionate communication of insight.

— GEORGE BERNARD SHAW

Our modern beliefs about sex are taught to us. They are the product of our upbringing, and they vary drastically from one culture to the next. However, our physiologic response to sexuality is a different matter. That comes from our instincts and is uniform throughout our species. The conflict between these two vastly different faces of sexuality provides a bountiful source of humor. The following series of lessons reflect human sexuality as portrayed by humorists.

The Lady in the Bar

A man walks into a bar and sees a pretty woman sitting by herself on a barstool.

He walks up to her and says, "Hi. How's it going?"

She turns to him, looks deep into his eyes, and says, "I'll screw anybody, anytime, anywhere, for any reason. My place, your place, anywhere you like, it doesn't matter."

He says, "No kidding! So what law firm are you with?"

This is a very intriguing joke. It is based on a homonym. Homonyms are pairs of words that have different meanings but are pronounced and spelled the same. They often have some common roots in their etymologies.

For example, consider the word *bank,* as in a riverbank but also as in a financial institution. These two words have the same root meaning. A bank was once a pile of stored resources, such as banked coal, firewood, or grain. The use of the word later diverged to mean a place where resources are kept for later use (financial institution) and also a sloping physical feature resembling a pile of material (riverbank). Homonyms reveal hidden relationships.

The "Lady in the Bar" exploits the conflict between two people who become lovers. The word *screw* is a homonym with several different meanings, all with some shared root. It is a slang word meaning to copulate or engage in sex. It is a mechanical device that can be forced into a round opening by twisting or turning. The same screw can use force and leverage to overcome resistance and cause changes in a system. However, *screw* also has sinister synonyms: cheat, defraud, deceive, victimize, dominate, take advantage of, and betray.

The root source of the term is the thumb screw, a device of torture used in the 16th century. It was a very effective device and a person exposed to a thumb screw was said to be screwed. Victims were completely dominated by the torturer and had no escape. In the 17th century, the word became associated with copulation and with other events that impacted a person in an inescapable, irreversible, negative fashion.

When two people become lovers, each often has hidden agendas. These may or may not be harmful to the other party. When lovers commit themselves to sex, they place themselves at considerable risk in terms of disease, reputation, financial obligations, pregnancy, physical injury, and personal conflict. The essential underlying truth is that a simple mundane event such as sex can have major undesirable irreversible life changing impact. Both parties in a sexual relationship put their social capital at risk, and both are vulnerable, naked, and exposed, to use other words that are common to both the bedroom and the courtroom.

A Sense of Humor

God told men they would find faithful and obedient wives in all the corners of the Earth. Then men discovered that God had made the Earth round, and God laughed and laughed.

This joke exploits the naïve expectations men have of women. Women are not naturally faithful and obedient to men. Rather, women manipulate men to their needs. There is a period in the life of a woman when she needs the support of men, but that is only when she has small children.

About 5000 years ago, men adopted a strategy of subjugating women, with variable success. Women are independent creatures with separate goals and strategies for survival.

The reader invariably assumes that God in this joke is male. It is funnier if read in the context of God being female.

The Book Store

A prospective husband in a bookstore asked the saleswoman, "Do you have a book called *Husband, the Master of the House?*"

The woman responded, "Yes, in the fiction and comics section on the first floor!"

Just another joke about an inexperienced man having unrealistic expectations of his relationship with his soon to be wife.

Problems at home

A man comes home to an empty house and finds a note on the refrigerator that says, "This is not working. I've taken the children and gone to my mother's house."

He opens the fridge, takes out a beer, and thinks, "The beer feels cold. I wonder why she thinks it's not working."

Men and women have very different concepts of what constitutes a home. Women think of the people in the home and their relationships, whereas men think of the physical structure and the stuff in it.

Becoming acquainted

Young Son: "Is it true, Dad, I heard that in some parts of Africa a man doesn't know his wife until he marries her?"

Dad: "That happens in every country, son."

Of course, this would work just as well if the gender was reversed. You never know anyone well until you have lived with them for a few years.

Who is in Charge?

Do you want to talk to the man in charge or the woman who knows what's going on?

This is a common expression, and persists because it reflects some truths. Women are generally more adept at grasping social relationships and have a better understanding of what is going on in an office, a business, or a family. They are also more aware of where things are located in a store or a home. Yet they are usually subservient to men for artificial reasons based on culture rather than expertise.

In Agreement

After a quarrel, a husband said to his wife, "You know, I was a fool when I married you."

She replied, "Yes, dear, but I was in love, and I didn't notice."

The essence of humor is reversal. This joke is an example of a power reversal, in which the dominant person in the story suddenly changes in the punch line. Usually it is the woman who comes out on top. It is a very common form in jokes about relationships and sex.

Of course, the truth is they were both fools when they married. That is the essence of being in love.

A Wedding Toast

A wedding toast: I would like the bride and groom to look at each other. You are now looking into the eyes of the person who is statistically most likely to murder you. To the bride and groom!

The Happy Husband

When a newly married man looks happy, we know why. But when a ten-year married man looks happy, we wonder why.

Silence

I once gave my husband the silent treatment for an entire week.
When it was over, he said, "We got along really well there for a while!"

Wife Wanted

A lonely man placed an ad in the paper.
"Wanted: A wife."
Within a week, he'd received hundreds of replies.
They were all the same: "You can have mine."

I Wonder Which One

When a married man opens the car door for his wife, it is either a new car or a new wife.

Thousands of jokes address the decay of romance that occurs over time as couples become intolerant of each other. They play upon the contrast between the myth of happily-ever-after and the reality of the post-romantic relationship. Recall Rodney Dangerfield's joke on the first page of this book.

Arizona Hitchhiker

Sally was driving home from one of her business trips in Northern Arizona when she saw an elderly Navajo woman walking on the side of the road. She stopped the car and asked the old woman if she wanted a ride.

With a silent nod of thanks, the woman got into the car. Resuming the journey, Sally tried in vain to make a bit of small talk with the Navajo woman. The old woman just sat silently, looking intently at everything she saw, studying every little detail until she noticed a brown bag on the seat next to Sally.

"What in the bag?" asked the old woman.

Sally looked down at the brown bag and said, "It's a bottle of wine. I got it for my husband."

The Navajo woman was silent for another moment or two. Then, speaking with the quiet wisdom of an elder, she said, "Good trade."

This is reputed to be a true story taken from Readers Digest decades ago. The Navajo have an ancient matrilineal, matrilocal family structure that persists today in rural areas. Women own everything and men are transient in their lives. To this elderly Navajo woman, it would be only natural to consider a husband a possession that could be traded for a bottle of wine.

The Joke is on the Butcher

Many years had passed since the embarrassing day when a young woman with a baby in her arms entered the butcher's shop. She confronted him with the news that the baby was his and asked what he would do about it. He offered to provide her with free meat until the boy was sixteen. She agreed.

He had been counting the years off on his calendar, and one day the teenager, who had been collecting the meat each week, came into the shop and said, "I'll be sixteen tomorrow."

"I know," said the butcher with a smile, "I've been counting too. Tell your mother, when you take this parcel of meat home, that it is the last free meat she'll get, and watch the expression on her face."

When the boy arrived home, he told his mother. The woman nodded and said, "Son, go back to the butcher and tell him I have also had free bread, free milk, and free produce for the last sixteen years, and watch the expression on his face!"

This is a great example of a power reversal joke. The young woman has outsmarted the butcher and several other men as well.

The story is reminiscent of the women in the Yanomami culture in the Amazon who acknowledge all their sexual partners during pregnancy as joint fathers of the child. The custom increases the resources women acquire for raising their children.

The underlying truth is that promiscuity can be financially rewarding if a woman plays her cards right.

Stolen Credit Cards

His wife's credit cards were stolen, but he chose not to report it because the thief was spending less money than she had.

The Boutique

A sign outside a women's clothing store reads, "Your husband called and said you can spend all the money you want."

Feeling Generous

A man is dressing in a busy locker room at the country club when a phone rings on the bench beside him. He answers and listens to the woman on the other end. After a moment, he says, "Well, if you like it, then I'm sure I'll like it too. We need a bigger house. Just offer them whatever they are asking."

After listening for a bit longer, he says, "Sure. You deserve a new car. I'm sure yours is out of style. Just pick out whatever you want and tell them I'll come by to pay for it."

He finishes the call with "Love you, too." Then turns to the room and shouts, "Does anyone know whose phone this is?"

Jokes about wives spending too much money have riled up some feminists. They feel such jokes promote the idea that women are dependent on men for money and that money belongs more to the man than the woman in a marriage. In fact, these jokes merely reflect the natural history of human child rearing strategies.

This is a good example of the conflict between our primitive emotions and our modern learned behaviors. Our biological nature dictates that, for the most part, men serve the role of supplying resources to women, and women use those resources to feed and nurture the family. It all goes back to the pelvis and the kneecap. Mothers of small children have historically been dependent on a mate to provide for them. That is how humans have survived since we learned to stand upright.

Today it is true that women also earn money and sometimes earn more than their husbands. The family money in a marriage indeed belongs to both partners. However those are recent political, legal, and social developments, and they apply to only a small segment of humanity. They do not change our instincts or basic human nature. If people had changed how they feel about wives using more resources than their husbands can provide, these jokes would be extinct.

The Difference between a Mistress, a Prostitute, and a Wife

The mistress lies on her back during sex and thinks, "Oh! Harder! Harder!"

The prostitute lies on her back and thinks, "Faster, faster …"

The wife lies on her back and thinks, "Beige. I think I'll paint the ceiling beige."

Here is an entirely plausible story of three women having sex for three different reasons, none of which have anything to do with reproduction. The first is intent on pleasure, the second is earning a living, and the third is simply satisfying a marital obligation. The truth is, humans have a lot of sex, and very little of it is for reproduction. The conflict lies in the wife's thoughts during coitus. Unlike the other two women, she is not thinking about sex at all, but about a mundane detail of the décor in her home. She is completely disinterested in the sex, but it keeps a roof over her head.

Man Rule

Size doesn't matter. All that matters is where you get to put it.

Here is an interesting joke that is not generally funny to women, but is to men, reflecting their different perspectives. Penis size does indeed matter to a woman for her pleasure (or discomfort), but to a man it only matters to the extent that it attracts women.

The primary objective for men is increased access to women, and there are many other factors, such as appearance, wealth, personality, timing, and a hundred other items of social capital that matter more than penis size. All that matters to a man's primitive instincts is access to vaginas, and penis size is of minor importance.

Being Practical

Dr. Goldstein was having dinner with his wife in a posh restaurant when a stunning young blonde approached him, said, "Hi, Sammy," kissed him, and then walked away.

Mrs. Goldstein was shocked and said, "Who was that?!"

The good doctor replied, "Oh. That was my mistress."

"You have a mistress?! How long has this been going on?"

"About three years," he answered.

"Well! This is outrageous!" she said. "I want a divorce!"

"No, you don't," he said. "Don't be silly. You've got it made. You don't have to work. Your kids are in private school. I buy you a new car every year. And I never ask you for sex. "

At that moment, a gorgeous redhead walked up and said, "Hi, Sammy," kissed him, and walked away.

His wife said, "OK, and who was that?"

The good doctor responded, "That was Dr. Thompson's mistress."

Mrs. Goldstein replied, "Oh. I think ours is prettier." And returned to eating her meal.

Notice how easily we buy into the premise of this story. Mrs. Goldstein's initial reaction to the mistress is based on her cultural belief that her husband should remain faithful. The pair bond these two once had is long gone. They are no longer in love. Their marriage is now a business partnership. She is afraid that the mistress will take her husband and her financial support.

Her fear vanishes once she is reassured that her lifestyle will continue without interruption. Her husband's mistress no longer threatens her. She not only accepts the mistress as another of their joint possessions but even expresses pride in the young woman's beauty. It is, after all, representative of her husband's financial success.

Note also that this is an example of polygyny.

The Jewelry Store

An older man walked into a jewelry store with a young woman. He told the jeweler he was looking for a special ring for his girl-friend. The jeweler looked through his stock and brought out a $5,000 ring. The man said, "No, I'd like to see something more special."

The jeweler went to his special stock and brought another ring over. "Here's a stunning ring at only $40,000," the jeweler said. The lady's eyes sparkled, and her whole body trembled with excitement.

Seeing this, the old man said, "We will take it."

The jeweler asked how payment would be made, and the man stated, "By check. I know you need to make sure my check is good, so I will write it now, and you can take it to the bank Monday to verify the funds. I will pick the ring up Monday afternoon."

On Monday morning the jeweler angrily phoned the old man and said, "Sir, there's no money in that account."

The old man said, "I know, but let me tell you what a weekend I had."

This story exploits the human female response to expensive gifts. The older man has learned to use that response to get what he wants from a young woman. From the beginning of time, human males have used gifts to obtain sexual services. Men use the promise of commitment and support to obtain sex, and it is an effective strategy.

The Lesson

A young lady came home from school and told her mother that today she learned how mommies get babies. Her mother was a little surprised but listened as the girl explained what her friend, Julie, had told her during school.

Julie told how she had peeked into her parents' bedroom and seen her mother and father naked on the bed. The mother kissed her father's "thing" and put it in her mouth over and over again until he shook all over.

"Oh no," said the girl's mother, "that's not how mommies get babies. That's how mommies get jewelry."

This is one out of hundreds of jokes exploiting this particular aspect of human sexuality. It is the other side of the story expressed in the previous joke. From the beginning of time, human females have used sex to obtain gifts. Women trade sexual services for support.

Scientific Fact

Scientists have discovered a food which eliminates a woman's desire for sex.

It's called wedding cake.

Women who are not financially secure are willing, even anxious, to give sex to men in trade for devotion and support. Once a woman enters into a standard Western marriage contract, her financial support is assured, and she loses her incentive to initiate, or even tolerate, sex.

This joke does not make sense in fundamentalist Muslim cultures and is not funny. In those cultures there is no premarital sex. Also, the marriage contract stipulates that sex is a wifely duty, and women may not refuse their husbands' advances.

Tradeoff

God said to Adam, "I have some good news and some bad."
Adam asked for the good news first.
God answered, "I'm giving you a brain and a penis."
"What's the bad news?" asked Adam.
God replied: "I'm only giving you enough blood for one of them to work at a time!"

Men become single-minded when sexually aroused and do not think clearly. They will foolishly make promises and commitments to women to obtain sex. Women instinctively know this and use their sexuality to get what they want. This is how women have survived and raised their children since the dawn of time.

Motivation

A homeowner got into his grubbiest clothes on Saturday morning and set about doing all the chores he'd been putting off for weeks. He'd cleaned out the garage, pruned the hedges, and was halfway through mowing the lawn when a woman pulled up in the driveway and yelled out the window, "Hey, what do you get for your yard work?"

The fellow thought for a minute, then answered, "The lady who lives here lets me sleep with her."

His answer is clever, unexpected, and true on several levels, all of which reflect a man's willingness to work for a woman in return for sex, whether as a laborer or a husband.

Jimmy Stewart's favorite joke

When Jimmy Stewart was asked to tell his all-time favorite joke, this was the story he told.

A married man was quietly reading a book when his wife approached him and asked, "If I died, would you remarry?"

The man replied, "Well, what kind of question is that? That's kind of morbid. Why would you even ask that?"

She persevered, "But would you remarry if I died?"

He responded, "Well, I'm still young and healthy, so yes, I guess I would remarry."

She continued, "Would she live in the house I live in?"

He said, "Well, it's a good house, and it's paid off, so I guess she would."

She asked, "Would she sleep in the bed I sleep in?"

He said, "It's a good bed, and there is no reason to change it, so I guess she would."

She asked, "Would she use my golf clubs?"

He said, "No, of course not. That's silly. She's left-handed."

Here is a wonderful bit of humor and gentle truth about a taboo subject. We never talk openly about it, but we all know humans constantly monitor for alternative mates. While the husband scolds his wife for asking such probing questions, in the end, he accidentally reveals that he does have a woman in mind to replace her if she were to die. It is a basic human behavior.

What Was the Question?

A human physiology lecturer notices that he is losing the attention of his class, so, to try to wake them up, he singles out a woman in the front row. He asks her, "Do you know what your asshole is doing when you're having an orgasm?"

She responds, "He's usually out playing golf with his buddies."

This is not the answer we expected, and it is rich with irony and revelations. She has orgasms when her male partner is absent from the house. She thinks of him when she hears the term asshole, indicating their pair-bond has expired. We are left to guess whether she is alone during her orgasms

Missing Out on the Fun

I asked my wife to let me know when she has an orgasm next time.

She said she doesn't like to bother me when I'm at work.

Just another comment on the same theme. Again, we are left to wonder whether she is alone at the time.

Wives' secrets

There is a rumor that lesbian relationships never last. This is not true. My girlfriend and I have been together for fifty years, and we are just as in love as the day we met. The key is never to let our husbands find out.

See how easy it is to accept the premise that women can be married to men, receiving the financial benefits of that relationship, yet obtaining an entirely different set of benefits from romantic relations with women. The success of jokes like these reveals our knowledge that the heterosexual population contains a lot of bisexual people.

This joke touches on another topic. Men are generally unaware of what women do when they are together. It is entirely credible that two women could have an affair stretching over decades without their husbands ever suspecting. When a woman is visiting with another woman, it never occurs to their husbands that they may be having sex.

Fantasy

You're the kind of girl I always imagine being with when I have sex with my husband.

Most bisexuals are in long-term heterosexual relationships. Women accuse husbands of fantasizing about someone else when making love, but wives do it too. In this case, the wife fantasizes about a woman, adding additional conflict and humor.

A Late-Night Surprise

Bubba is walking home from the bar late one night and sees the outline of a woman in the shadows. "Twenty dollars," she whispers.

Bubba had never been with a hooker before and decides, what the hell, it's only twenty bucks. So, he goes into the bushes and joins her.

They're "engaged" for a few minutes when, all of a sudden, a light flashes on them. It is a police officer. "What's going on here?" asks the officer.

"I'm making love to my wife!" Bubba answers, sounding annoyed.

"Oh, I'm sorry," says the cop, "I didn't know."

"Well, neither did I, 'til ya shined that light in her face."

Here are a husband and wife whose pair bond has ended. Both are straying. He is trading money for sex, and she trades sex for money. He is annoyed to discover the woman is actually his wife. We are left to assume that she was equally surprised.

It is funny because there are multiple surprises and conflicts at once. Suddenly, he is not physically cheating on his wife (but he is in spirit), and his wife is not cheating on him (except in spirit). They are just spouses having sex, so why is he annoyed? Is it because this changes their relationship, or is it a disappointment because nothing has changed except that she has his twenty dollars?

The underlying truth in this joke is that there can be a very fine line between the post-romantic relationship and frank prostitution.

A temporary arrangement

A physician reviewed the answers to questionnaires filled out by his new patients, Mr. and Mrs. Thompson. He noticed that Mr. Thompson reported having sex twice a week, while his wife said she has sex three times a night. When he asked them about this discrepancy, the husband explained, "Oh, that's just until we get the second mortgage paid off."

This is just another joke about a woman using sex to obtain resources, but in this case, her husband is in on the scheme. This is a reversal of the joke about Mrs. Goldstein's response to Dr. Goldstein's mistress. Here, the husband has cast aside the standard taboo on extramarital sex by his spouse. He is not threatened as long as she is just doing it for the money and sharing her earnings with him.

Relax

A woman is relaxing in bed with a man when the phone rings. She gets up and answers it, then returns to her lover. He asks, "Who was that?"

She answers, "It was my husband."

He asks, "Should I be leaving?"

She responds, "No, you can relax and stay a while. He told me he is playing poker with you."

Hundreds of jokes exploit the mutual betrayal in marriages when both partners cheat. A philandering man is failing to guard his own mate against interlopers. Seeking sexual pleasure outside the marriage is human nature, and the risks are well known.

This is another power reversal joke in which the woman is smarter than her husband.

Weee bit

A wealthy and extraordinarily handsome young man decided he had a responsibility to marry the perfect woman so they could produce beautiful children beyond comparison. With that as his mission, he began searching for the perfect wife. Shortly after that, he met a farmer who had three stunning daughters who positively took his breath away.

He explained his mission to the farmer, asking for permission to marry one of them. The farmer simply replied, "They're lookin' to get married, so you came to the right place. Look 'em over and pick the one you want." The man had a date with the first daughter. The next day, the farmer asked for his opinion.

"Well," said the man, "she's just a weeeeee bit ... not that you can hardly notice ... pigeon-toed." The farmer nodded and suggested the man date one of the other girls, so the man went out with the second daughter. The next day, the farmer again asked how things went.

"Well," the man replied, "she's just a weeeee bit ... not that you can hardly tell ... cross-eyed." The farmer nodded and suggested he date the third girl to see if things might be better. So, he did.

The next morning, the man rushed in, exclaiming, "She's perfect, just perfect. She's the one I want to marry." So, they were wed right away, and in no time at all, they were expecting a child. Months later, the baby was born. When the man visited the nursery, he was horrified: the baby was the ugliest, most pathetic human you can imagine. He rushed to his father-in-law, asking how such a thing could happen, considering the parents' beauty.

"Well," explained the farmer, "when you met her, she was just a weeeee bit ... not that you could hardly tell ... pregnant."

This is another example of power reversal. The farmer and his daughters have outsmarted a person of higher rank. This arrogant young man has suffered a sudden reversal of fortunes at the hands of his father-in-law, his wife, and her two sisters. He judged these three young women based only on their physical beauty, remaining completely oblivious to matters of much greater importance. His superficial assessment made it easy for his future in-laws to manipulate him into marrying the girl who was already pregnant. Now, he has been cuckolded.

Outward Appearance

Marrying someone for their good looks is like buying a house for the paint color.

This is a more concise version of the prior joke, addressing the folly of choosing a marital partner based only on physical beauty.

Who's Your Daddy

One Sunday morning, William burst into the living room and said, "Dad! Mom! I have some great news for you! I am getting married to the most beautiful girl in town. She lives a block away, and her name is Susan."

After dinner, William's dad took him aside. "Son, I have to talk with you. Your mother and I have been married for thirty years. She's a wonderful wife, but she has never offered much excitement in the bedroom, so I used to fool around with women a lot. Susan is actually your half-sister, and I'm afraid you can't marry her."

William was heartbroken. After eight months, he eventually started dating girls again. A year later, he came home and very proudly announced, "Diane said yes! We're getting married in June."

Again, his father insisted on a private conversation and broke the sad news. "Diane is your half-sister too, William. I'm awfully sorry about this."

William was furious! He finally decided to go to his mother with the news.

"Dad has done so much harm. I guess I'm never going to get married," he complained. "Every time I fall in love, Dad tells me the girl is my half-sister."

His mother just shook her head. "Don't pay any attention to what he says, dear. He's not your real father."

We find this humorous because we know paternal discrepancy is a two-edged sword. The philandering male is not at home guarding his mate. Women are just as likely as men to engage in infidelity.

There is a certain satisfaction in seeing the tables turned on the father, who was so critical of his wife. He believes he has cuckolded other men, but he was cuckolded.

The Maid Gets a Raise

The maid asked for a raise.

The Madam was very upset and asked, "Now Maria, why do you think you deserve a raise?"

"Well, Madam," she answered, "there are three reasons. The first is that I iron better than you do."

Madam asked, "Who said you iron better than I do?"

Maria answered, "The Master said so."

Madam said, "Oh,"

The maid said, "The second reason is that I cook better than you do."

"Nonsense!" said the Madam. "Who told you that you cook better than I do?"

"The Master." answered the maid.

Madam responded, "Oh."

Maria went on, "And the third reason is that I am a better lover than you."

The Madam, now very upset, asked, "And did the Master say this as well?"

The maid answered, "No, Madam. The gardener did."

The maid got a raise.

Sexuality permeates all aspects of human life, including the workplace. It is entirely plausible that both the maid and the Madam have been having sex with the gardener. The gardener told the maid, and now the Madam is screwed.

This is another power reversal. In many sexual jokes, the woman outsmarts the man in the punch line. In this example, the subservient maid outsmarts the Madam of the house.

Sex with a Ghost

A professor at a major university is giving a lecture on the supernatural. To get a feel for his audience, he asks, "How many people here believe in ghosts?"

About 90 students raise their hands.

"Well, that's a good start," he says. "How many of you have seen a ghost?"

About 40 students raise their hands.

"That's good. Has anyone here ever talked to a ghost?"

About 15 students indicated they had.

"OK. Has anyone ever touched a ghost?"

Three students raise their hands.

"That's fantastic." He says. "Now, let me ask one more question. Has anyone ever had sex with a ghost?"

All the way in the back of the auditorium, Bubba raises his hand.

The professor takes off his glasses and says, "Son, in all the years that I have given this lecture, I have never met anyone who had sex with a ghost. Come down here and tell us about it."

The big redneck student replies with a nod and a grin and walks down to the podium. The professor asks, "So tell us, what is it like to have sex with a ghost?"

Bubba replies, "Shucks, from way back there, I thought you said goats."

Here is another example of an outlandish but plausible, conflicting reality. Human males are hyper-sexual and not very selective in their choice of sexual partners. They are quite capable of having sex with animals.

In 2010, an incident in Washington State made national news (Clarridge, 2010). Douglas Spink, a farm owner, ran a successful bed and breakfast that specialized in providing animals for sexual purposes. When the nature of his business was discovered by the authorities, he was arrested, and the ASPCA confiscated his animals.

However, it was unclear whether he had broken any laws. It is illegal to engage in prostitution in Washington State, and it is illegal to procure prostitutes for others. It is also illegal to engage in sex with animals. However, there is no specific law against prostituting animals. Mr. Spink was eventually charged with animal cruelty, although there was no evidence that the animals were harmed.

Hundreds of jokes play on this aspect of human sexuality, whether it concerns sex with animals, inanimate objects, garden vegetables, mechanical devices, or even ghosts.

Succinct

What do you call a man who marries another man?
A priest.

These short jokes often carry more significance than is immediately evident. Homosexual relations between men conflict with the chaste reputation of priests, creating humor.

However, there is a profound underlying truth. A man who marries another man is free from the burden of providing for a family. In the more general sense of the word "priest," he is able to be a learned man, scholar, philosopher, naturalist, scientist, mathematician, teacher, and holy man."

Sex for a Nun

How do you get a nun pregnant? You dress her as an altar boy.

It is difficult to find a good joke about homosexuality in the Catholic priesthood that does not exploit pedophilia, which is unfortunate.

For many years, the Catholic Church refused to acknowledge their pedophiles in order to hide clerical homosexuality from the public. This suggested that the church condones pedophilia and, by extension, that all homosexual males are pedophiles. However, the belief that homosexual men are more inclined than heterosexual men to engage in pedophilia has been repeatedly disproven. Heterosexual men abuse female children at about the same rate that homosexual men abuse male children.

Pedophilia and homosexuality are two entirely separate issues. It is only in the politics of the church that they have become linked. Pedophilia, whether hetero- or homosexual, is a despicable crime against children. However, homosexuality is a more complex matter. It is a normal variant of human sexual behavior and has played a vital role in advancing human culture, particularly Western cultures and Christianity.

Nonetheless, jokes on this subject reveal the public knowledge that homosexuality is widespread in the Catholic Church and that pedophilia is an established problem in some parishes.

Who's who

How do you tell which priests are gay?
The gay priests end their prayers with the words, "Ah. Men."

This joke is based on a homophone, a pair of words that sound the same but have different spellings and meanings. It elicits mirth because the first line suggests a useful answer, but "Ah, men" and "Amen" sound the same, so the answer is of no help. We know many priests are gay, and there is no simple way to know which ones. This joke suggests the possibility they are all gay.

You Misunderstand Me

A nun went to a psychologist and complained, "Doctor, young women keep coming to me for emotional support, and I keep taking advantage of them sexually. I feel so guilty."

He said, "Certainly, with a few weeks of therapy, we can help you gain much more self-control."

She responded, "Forget that! I just want to stop feeling guilty."

This is just a reminder that homosexuality and sexual exploitation of parishioners are not limited to male clerics.

The Comeback

Suzanne Westenhoefer is a lesbian comedian who performs for heterosexual crowds. She once had the following interaction with a heckler. He shouted, "Hey, did you get that way because you had some kind of a bad sexual relationship with a guy?"

She responded, "Yeah – like if that's all it took, the entire female population would be gay, sir, and I'd be up here talking about the weather, all right."

For men, any sex that ends in an orgasm without an injury is good. Sex is its own reward. Women, however, engage in a lot of sex with men that is not for the women's pleasure. The female incentives for sex are much more diverse. Women have many ulterior motives for sex. It is a device to manipulate men, and it is, for the most part, a chore. In that context, all women experience many "bad sexual relationships" with men.

Good illustrative jokes about the LGBTQ community are more difficult to document than jokes about heterosexuality for several reasons. First and foremost, jokes exploiting the LGBTQ community have become taboo in the past few decades, at least for heterosexual comedians. They remain fair game only if the comedian is gay. Second, the main genre is now stand-up comedy rather than text, and it often does not translate well to the written page. Third, most jokes about homosexuality are not actually about sex.

The great majority of gay and lesbian jokes are about the cultural and social aspects of the non-heterosexual community. There are only so many jokes that can be told about oral and anal sex, and they quickly become tedious. Many others deal with "coming out," but these also exhaust the subject and become tiresome.

The most enlightening jokes are those told by homosexuals to homosexuals. Heterosexuals who are not in the culture do not understand the premises of the joke or see the humor. Likewise, jokes told by homosexuals about heterosexuals are revealing but are often opaque to heterosexual listeners (Flowers, 1995; Nardi, 2003; Overstreet, 2021).

Underachievers

Women who wish to prove that they are as good as men in bed lack ambition.

Sex between women is very different from heterosexual sex. Sex with men is primarily motivated by the male desire for an orgasm and typically ends with that event long before the woman's needs are satisfied. Sex between women is a social interaction motivated by the emotional needs of the women, and it may last for hours.

Another light bulb joke

How many lesbians does it take to screw in a light bulb?

One to change the bulb, three to bring the pot-luck dinner, and three to make the self-empowering documentary.

The reader expects a punch line about sex, but this is a joke about civil rights and female independence from male domination. Many women feel oppressed by the patriarchal Western family structure, the so-called nuclear family. To these women, every time a woman performs a "man's job," it is a call for celebration, heraldry, and documentation.

Baggage

What does a lesbian bring to a second date? A U-Haul.

Here is a good example of an inside joke in the lesbian community. The obvious interpretation is that lesbians co-habitat after brief relationships. However, there is more to it than that. The joke refers to the emotional baggage that appears on subsequent dates. It is also a nod to lesbian self-reliance. They are inclined to move their stuff themselves rather than hire men to do it.

Breeders

What do breeders do for foreplay? They take off their underwear.
How do breeders have sex? Yuck! Who cares?!

Lesbians have a category of derogatory jokes specifically directed at heterosexual women with children, referred to as "breeders."

Lesbian sex is a drawn-out romantic exercise that may last for hours. It is not driven forward by the male urgency to achieve ejaculation. Women having sex with women can take their time and enjoy each other's company. Sex between heterosexual couples is often ruined by the man's desire to get to the endpoint, yet the women tolerate it. Not surprisingly, lesbians have a low opinion of heterosexual sex and heterosexual women.

There are, of course, thousands of other jokes that are told about human sexuality, and each of them has a message. Together, they reveal the true nature of human beings. They have to because otherwise, they would not be funny, and they would not be propagated by the public. When you see or hear a good joke about human sexuality, look for the truth it reveals.

Humor is the good-natured side of truth.

— MARK TWAIN

BIBLIOGRAPHY

Adams, C. (2007, October 19). Who's your daddy? Is it true 10-15 % of children in modern society were not sired by their putative fathers? *The Straight Dope.* http://www.straightdope.com

Adovasio, J. M., Page, J., & Soffer, O. (2007). *The invisible sex: Uncovering the true roles of women in prehistory.* New York, NY: HarperCollins Publishers.

Ahrons, C. R. (1994). *The good divorce.* New York, NY: HarperCollins Publishers.

Ainsworth, C. (2018, October 22). Sex Redefined: The Idea of 2 Sexes Is Overly Simplistic. *Nature.* https://www.scientificamerican.com/article/sex-redefined-the-idea-of-2-sexes-is-overly-simplistic1/

Ames, A., Burke, D., & Ellis, L. (1987, December). Sexual Orientation as a continuous variable: A comparison between the sexes. *Archives of Sexual Behavior, 16* (6), 523-529. Doi: 10.1007/BF01541716

Anderson, K. G. (2006). How well does paternity confidence match actual paternity? Evidence from worldwide paternity rates. *Current Anthropology 47* (3), 513-521.

Armstrong, K. (1994). *A History of God: The 4,000-year quest of Judaism, Christianity and Islam.* New York, NY: Ballantine Books.

An arrangement of marriages. (1993, January 1). *Psychology Today.* http://www.psychologytoday.com

Aubuchon, V. (2010). *World population growth history.* http://www.vaughns-1-pagers.com

Ayres, B. D. (1991, November 21). Fertility doctor accused of fraud. *The New York Times.* http://www.nytimes.com

Badgett, M. L., & Sears, B. (2004). *Same-sex couples and same-sex couples raising children in California: Data from Census 2000.* http://repositories.cdlib.org/uclalaw/williams/census/california.2000

Bailey, J. M., Keller, M. C., Macgregor, S., Martin, N. G., Morley, K. I., Shekar, S. N. & Zietsch, B. P. (2008, July 1). Genetic factors predisposing to homosexuality may increase mating success in heterosexuals. *Evolution and Human Behavior, 29,* 424-433. Doi: 10.1016/j.evolhumbehav.2008.07.002

Baker, J. A., Fox, C. A., & Wolf, H. S. (1970). Measurement of intra-vaginal and intra-uterine pressures during human coitus by radio-telemetry. *Journal of the Society for Reproduction and Fertility, 22,* 243-251.

Baker, R. (1996). *Sperm wars.* New York, NY: Perseus Books Group.

Bancroft, J. (2005). The endocrinology of sexual arousal. *Journal of Endocrinology, 186,* 411-427. doi: 10.1677/joe.1.06233

Barash, D. P. (n.d.). *Deflating the myth of monogamy.* http://www.trinity.edu/rnadeau/fys/barash%20on%20monogamy.htm

Batt, J., Hall, S., Hendricks, C., & Olson, D. (1998). *Gender differences in physical attraction*. http://www.units.muohio.edu/psybersite/attraction/gender.shtml

Battles, M. (2004). *Library: An Unquiet History*. New York, NY: W. W. Norton and Company, Inc.

Baumeister, R. F., & Vohs, K. D. (2004). Sexual economics: Sex as female resource for social exchange in heterosexual interactions. *Personality and Social Psychology Review, 8* (4), 339-363.

Beach, F. A., & Ford, C. S. (1951). *Patterns of sexual behavior*. New York, NY: Harper and Row.

Beil, D., Deininger, H., Kunz, G., Leyendecker, G., & Wildt, L. (1996). The dynamics of rapid sperm transport through the female genital tract: Evidence from vaginal sonography of uterine peristalsis and hysterosalpingoscintigraphy. *Human Reproduction, 11*(3), 627-632.

Bellis, MA., Hughes, K., Hughes, S., Ashton, JR. (2022, April 21). Measuring paternal discrepancy and its public health consequences. https://jech.bmj.com/content/59/9/749.short

Ben-Zeev, A. (2008, September 12). *When do we fall in love?* [Web log message]. http://www.psychologytoday.com/blog/in-the-name-love/200809/when-do-we-fall-in-love

Besl, J. (n.d.). *Births to unmarried moms increase sharply* [Web log message]. http://crcblog.typepad.com/crcblog/births-to-unmarried-moms-increase-sharply.html

Bing, J. M., Heller, D. (2003). How many lesbians does it take to screw in a light bulb? English *Faculty Publications, 3*. https://digitalcommons.odu.edu/English_fac_pubs/3

Blomberg, S. P., Kaplan, G., MacFarlane, G. R., & Rogers, L. J. (2007). Same-sex sexual behavior in birds: Expression is related to social mating system and state of development at hatching. *Behavioral Ecology, 18*, 21-33. Doi 10.1093/beheco/arl065

Blumberg, S. L., Markman, H. J., & Stanley, S. M. (2001). *Fighting for your marriage*. San Francisco, CA: John Wiley and Sons, Inc.

Boswell, J. (1995). *Same sex unions in pre-modern Europe*. New York, NY: Random House.

Brizendine, L. (2006). *The Female Brain*. New York, NY: Harmony Books.

Brizendine, L. (2010). *The Male Brain*. New York, NY: Harmony Books.

Brodman, J. Z. (2017). *Sex rules: Astonishing sexual practices and gender roles around the world*. Coral Gables, FL: Mango Publishing Group

Brooke, J. (2011, March 17). Did feminism cause divorce? *Huffington Post*. http://www.huffingtonpost.com

Brooks, M., Chiafari, F. A., Houtz, T., & Wenk, R. E. (1992). How frequent is heteropaternal superfecundation? *Acta Genet Med Gemellol (Roma), 41*(1), 43-47. http://www.ncbi.nlm.nih.gov/pubmed/1488855

Brown, A. (n.d.). *George Sand: An amazing woman*. Retrieved from http://www.amybrown.net/women/george.html

Browne, J. (2006). *Dating for Dummies* (2nd ed.). Hoboken, NJ: John Wiley and Sons.

Browning, D. (1989, October 11). Rethinking homosexuality. *The Christian Century*, 911-916. http://www.religion-online.org

Buss, D. M. (1985, January/February). Human mate selection. *American Scientist, 73,* 47-51.

Buss, D. M. (1989). Sex differences in human mate preferences: Evolutionary hypotheses tested in 37 cultures. *Behavioral and Brain Sciences, 12,* 1-49.

Buss, D. M. (2003). *The evolution of desire.* New York, NY: Perseus Books Group.

Buss, D. M., & Meston, C. M. (2007). *Why humans have sex.* Available from Archives of Sexual Behavior. (UMI no. 36: 477 – 507). Doi 10.1007/s10508-007-9175-2

Buss, D. M., & Schmitt, D. P. (1993). Sexual strategies theory: An evolutionary perspective on human mating. *Psychological Review 100*(2), 204-232.

Cacioppo, J. T., & Patrick, W. (2009). *Loneliness: Human nature and the need for social connection.* New York, NY: W. W. Norton & Company.

Caldwell, J. C., & Caldwell, P. (1990, May). High fertility in Sub-Saharan Africa. *Scientific American, 262*(5), 118-125.

Canfora, L. (1990). *The vanished library: A wonder of the ancient world.* Berkeley: University of California Press.

Cecil Jacobson. (2012, January 10). In *Wikipedia.* http://en.wikipedia.org/wiki/Cecil_-Jacobson

Cecil B. Jacobson [encyclopedia article]. (n.d.). In *NationMaster.* http://www.nationmaster.com/encyclopedia/Cecil-Jacobson

Census reports more than 130,000 same-sex couples say they're married. (2011, September 28). *Associated Press.* http://www.foxnews.com

Center for Gender Sanity. (2001, August 16). *Diagram of sex and gender.* http://gendersanity.com/diagram.shtml

Chandra, A., Copen, C., Mosher, W. D., & Sionean, C. (2011). Sexual behavior, sexual attraction, and sexual identity in the United States: Data from the 2006-2008 National Survey of Family Growth. *National Health Statistics Reports; no 36.* Hyattsville, MD: National Center for Health Statistics.

Charlton, B. M. (2018, March 12). *Bisexual teens five times more likely to become pregnant.* https://www.healio.com/news/pediatrics/20180312/bisexual-teens-five-times-more-likely-to-become-pregnant

Childfree. (2010, July 20). In *Wikipedia.* http://en.wikipedia.org/wiki/Childfree

Child Marriage in the United States. (2021, January 6). In *Wikipedia.* https://en.wikipedia.org/w/index.php?title=Child_marriage_in_the_United_States&action=history

Circumcision Information and Research Pages. (2008, August 9). *Foreskin sexual function/circumcision sexual dysfunction.* http://www.cirp.org/library/sex_function/

Clarridge, C. (2010, July 16). Man who ran animal-sex operation sentenced for probation violation. Seattle Times. Retrieved from https://www.seattletimes.com/seattle-news/man-who-ran-animal-sex-operation-sentenced-for-probation-violation/

Code of Hammurabi. (L. W. King, trans.). http://www.fordham.edu/halsall/ancient/hamcode.asp#horne

Cohen, K. M., & Savin-Williams, R. C. (2010, November 16). Can men have sex with men and still call themselves straight? *The Good Men Project.* http://www.alternet.org/story/148876/

Cohn, D. (2011). *Census Bureau: Flaws in same-sex couple data.* http://www.pewsocial-trends.org/2011/09/27/census-bureau-flaws-in-same-sex-couple-data/

Cohn, D. (2011). *How accurate are counts of same-sex couples?* http://www.pewsocialtrend-s.org/2011/08/25/how-accurate-are-counts-of-same-sex-couples/

Cohn, D., & Livingston, G. (2010). *More women without children.* http://pewre-search.org/pubs/1642/more-women-without-children

Cohn, D., Livingston, G., Passel, J. S., & Wang, W. (2011). *Barely half of U.S. adults are married—a record low: New marriages down 5% from 2009 to 2010.* www.pewsocial-trends.org/2011/12/14/barely-half-of-u-s-adults-are-married-a-record-low/

Coleman, E. (1985, Spring). Bisexual women in marriages. *Journal of Homosexuality, 11* (1-2), 87-99. http://www.ncbi.nlm.nih.gov/pubmed

Coontz, S. (2006). *Marriage, a history.* New York, NY: Penguin Group.

Copeland, P., & Hamer, D. (1994). *The science of desire: The search for the gay gene and the biology of behavior.* New York, NY: Simon & Schuster.

Davis, J. L. (2001, November 12). *What's so great about kissing?* http://www.medicinenet.-com/script/main/art.asp?articlekey=51171

Dawkins, R. (1989). *The selfish gene.* New York, NY: Oxford University Press.

Dawkins, R. (2006). *The God delusion.* New York, NY: Houghton Mifflin Company.

Dawood, K., & Puts, D. A. (2006, June). The evolution of female orgasm: Adaption or byproduct? *Twin Research and Human Genetics, 9*(3), 467-472.

de Waal, F. (1995). Bonobo sex and society. *Scientific American, 272*(3), 82-89.

de Waal, F. (1995). *Our inner ape.* New York, NY: Penguin Group.

Denig, E. T. (1989). *Five Indian tribes of the upper Missouri.* Norman: University of Oklahoma Press.

Diamant, A.L., Lever, J., McGuigan, K., & Schuster, M.A. (1999, December 13/27). Lesbians' sexual history with men: Implications for taking a sexual history. *Archives of Internal Medicine, 159,* 2730-2736.

Diamond, J. (1993). *The third chimpanzee.* New York, NY: HarperCollins Publishers.

Diamond, J. (1999). *Guns, germs, and steel: The fates of human societies.* New York, NY: W. W. Norton & Company.

Durante, K. M., & Li, N. P. (2009, April 23). Oestradiol level and opportunistic mating in women. *Biology Letters, 5*(2), 179-182.

Economist. (2004, February 12). *I get a kick out of you.* Retrieved from oxytocin.org website: http://www.oxytocin.org/oxytoc/love-science.html

Elton, C. (2009, November 18). Female sexual dysfunction: Myth or malady? *Time.* http://www.time.com

Emlen, D. (1997, November). Alternative reproductive tactics and male dimorphism in the horned beetle Onthophagus acuminatus (Coleoptera: Scarabaeidae). *Behavioral Ecology and Sociobiology, 41*(5), 335-341.

Engels, Meredith. (2015, May). Gay, bisexual teens more likely to get pregnant than straight peers: study. In *New York Daily News.* https://www.nydailynews.com/life-style/health/gay-bisexual-teens-pregnant-study-article-1.2226423

Enserink, M. (2005, June). Let's talk about sex and drugs. *Science, 308*(5728), 578.

Etcoff, N. (2000). *Survival of the prettiest: The science of beauty.* New York, NY: Anchor Books.

Fausto-Sterling, A. (1993, March/April). The five sexes: Why male and female are not enough. *The Sciences,* 20-24.

Fein, E. & Schneider, S. (2007). *All the rules: Time-tested secrets for capturing the heart of Mr. Right.* New York, NY: Hatchet Book Group USA.

Fertility sparks 'male rivalry'. (2006, April 25). *BBC News World Edition.* http://news.bbc.co.uk

Fielding, W. J. (1942). *Strange customs of courtship and marriage.* Philadelphia, PA: The Blakiston Company.

Finkel, E. J., Gable, S. L., Impett, E. A., & Strachman, A. (2008). Maintaining sexual desire in intimate relationships: The importance of approach goals. *Journal of Personality and Social Psychiatry, 94*(5), 808-823. Doi: 10.1037/0022-3514.94.5.808

Fisher, H. (1994). *Anatomy of love: A natural history of mating, marriage, and why we stray.* New York, NY: Random House Publishing Group.

Flowers, C. (1995). *Out, loud, and laughing: A collection of gay and lesbian Humor.* New York, NY: Doubleday.

Frank, P. W. (1981). A condition for sessile strategy. *The American Naturalist, 118,* 288-290.

Franklin, B. (1745). Advice to a Friend on Choosing a Mistress. Wikipedia. https://en.wikipedia.org/wiki/Advice_to_a_Friend_on_Choosing_a_Mistress

Fry, R., Kochhar, R., & Taylor, P. (2011, July 26). *Wealth gaps widen to record highs between whites, blacks and Hispanics.* http://pewsocialtrends.org/2011/07/26/wealth-gaps-rise-to-record-highs-between-whites-blacks-hispanics/

Laumann, E. O., et al. (1994). *Sex in America: A definitive survey.* New York, NY: Warner Books.

Laumann, E. O., et al. (1994). *The social organization of sexuality: Sexual practices in the United States.* Chicago, IL: University of Chicago Press.

Gangestad, S. W., & Simpson, J. A. (2000). The evolution of human mating: Trade-offs and strategic pluralism. *Behavioral and Brain Sciences, 23,* 573-644.

Gangestad, S. W., Garver-Apgar, C. E., & Thornhill, R. (2005). Women's sexual interests across the ovulatory cycle depend on primary partner developmental instability. *Proceedings of the Royal Society B, 272,* 2023-2027. Doi 10.1098/rspb.2005.3112

Garcia, J. R., Lloyd, E. A., Wallen, K., & Fisher, H. E. (2014, August 18). Variation in orgasm occurrence by sexual orientation in a sample of U.S. singles. *The Journal of Sexual Medicine.* https://doi.org/10.1111/jsm.12669

Gender wars: A peace plan. (2009, October 1). *Psychology Today.* http://www.psychologytoday.com

George Sand. (2010, May 9). In *Wikipedia.* http://en.wikipedia.org/wiki/George_Sand

Gilding, M. (2009). Paternity uncertainty and evolutionary psychology: How a seemingly capricious occurrence fails to follow laws of greater generality. *Sociology, 43*(1), 140-157. Doi: 10.1 177/0038038508099102

Gilding, M. (n.d.). *Using sex surveys to calculate the extent of paternal discrepancy.* http://www.tasa.org.au/conferences/conferencepapers07/papers/17.pdf

Gleick, J. (2011, May). Have meme, will travel. *Smithsonian, 43*(2), 88-94.

Goldstein, J. S. (2001). *War and gender: How gender shapes the war system and vice versa.* Cambridge, England. Cambridge University Press.

Goodstein, D. (1994, September 19). *The Big Crunch.* Paper presented at the National Conference on the Advancement of Research 48 Symposium, Portland, OR.

Gottman, J. M. (1995). *Why marriages succeed or fail.* New York, NY: Simon and Schuster.

Gottman, J. M., & Silver, N. (1999). *The seven principles for making marriage work.* New York, NY: Three Rivers Press.

Greenberg, D. (1990). *The construction of homosexuality.* Chicago, IL: University of Chicago Press.

Griffith, S. C., Owens, I. P., & Thuman, K. A. (2002). Extra pair paternity in birds: A review of interspecific variation and adaptive function. *Molecular Ecology, 11,* 2195-2212.

Guthrie, S. L. (2001). *Empiricism, naturalism, and theism.* http://www.sguthrie.net/empiricism.htm

Hamilton, B. E., Kirmeyer, S., Martin, J. A., Mathews, T. J., Menacker, F., Sutton, P. D., & Ventura, S. J. (2009, January 7). Births: Final data for 2006. *National Vital Statistics Reports, 57*(7), 1-13.

Harrell, S. (1997). *Human families.* Boulder, CO: Westview Press.

Harrison, J. R. (2003). *The nitrogen cycle: Of microbes and men.* http://www.visionlearning.com/library/module_viewer.php?mid=98

Haslam, N. (1997, October). Evidence that male sexual orientation is a matter of degree. *Journal of Personality and Social Psychology, 73*(4), 862-870. http://www.ncbi.nlm.nih.gov/pubmed/

Hawley, J. S., & Narayanan, V. (Eds.). (2006). *The life of Hinduism.* Berkeley: University of California Press.

Hayden, T., & Potts, M. (2010). *Sex and war: How biology explains warfare and terrorism and offers a path to a safer world.* Dallas, TX: Benbella Books.

Heine, K. (2005, November 1). *A little perspective on marriage.* http://www.azcentral.com/families/articles/1101marriageevolution01.html

Heterosexual-homosexual continuum. (2010, March 18). In *Wikipedia.* http://en.wikipedia.org/wiki/Heterosexual-homosexual_continuum

Heussner, K. M. (2010, July 8). Addicted to love? It's not you, it's your brain: Recovering from heartbreak is like kicking a drug addiction, study says. *ABC News.* http://www.abcnews.go.com

High hormone levels in women may lead to infidelity, study shows. (2009, January 30). *Science Daily.* http://www.sciencedaily.com/releases/2009/01/090127133113.htm

Hinde, R. A. (1999). *Why gods persist.* New York, NY: Routledge.

Hinsch, B. (1990). *Passions of the cut sleeve: The male homosexual tradition in China.* New York, NY: Reed Business Information, Inc.

History of male circumcision. (2010, September 30). In *Wikipedia.* http://en.wikipedia.org/wiki/History_of_male_circumcision

Hitchens, C., & Hitchens, P. (2010, October 12). *Can civilization survive without God?*

Debate hosted by Pew Forum on Religion and Public Life. http://pewresearch.org/pubs/1785/hitchens-brothers-debate-does-civilization-need-religion

Hite, S. (2004). *The Hite report: A nationwide study of female sexuality.* New York, NY: Seven Stories Press. (Original work published in 1976)

Homma, Y., Poon, C. S., Saewyc, E. M., & Skay, C. L. (2008). Stigma management? The links between enacted stigma and teen pregnancy trends among gay, lesbian, and bisexual students in British Columbia. *Canadian Journal of Human Sexuality, 17*(3), 123-139. http://www.ncbi.nlm.nih.gov

Homosexual behavior in animals. (2009, May 19). In *Wikipedia.* http://en.wikipedia.org/wiki/Homosexuality_in_animals

Hooper, J. (2010, September 17). Pope's visit: Benedict tells politicians that religion is being marginalized. *The Guardian.* http://www.guardian.co.uk

Horne, C. F. (1915). The *Code of Hammurabi: An introduction.* http://www.fordham.edu/halsall/ancient/hamcode.asp#horne

Hrdy, S. B. (2000, April). The optimal number of fathers: Evolution, demography, and history in the shaping of female mate preferences. *Annals of the New York Academy of Sciences, 907*, 75-96.

Human-animal marriage. (2010, November 18). In *Wikipedia.* http://en.wikipedia.org/wiki/Human-animal_marriage

Italie, L. (2010, May 6). Study: Older, unmarried, educated moms on the rise. *Huffington Post.* http://www.huffingtonpost.com

Jahme, C. (2010, May 6). Penis size: An evolutionary perspective. *The Guardian.* http://www.guardian.co.uk

James, B. (1994, September 8). Overpopulation has a brief history. *The New York Times.* http://www.nytimes.com

Janssen, D. F. (2002, October). Aboriginal Australia. In *Growing Up Sexually. Volume I: World Reference Atlas.* http://www2.hu-berlin.de/sexology/GESUND/ARCHIV/GUS/AUSTRALIAOLD.HTM

Jetha, C., & Ryan, C. (2010). *Sex at dawn: The prehistoric origins of modern sexuality.* New York, NY: Harper Collins Publishers.

Johns, C. H. (1910). Babylonian law—The Code of Hammurabi. In *The Encyclopedia Britannica* (11th ed.). New York City, NY: Encyclopaedia Britannica Inc.

Johnson, R. A. (1977). *SHE: Understanding feminine psychology.* New York, NY: Harper and Row.

Jones, S. L. (2002, June 22). Sexual script theory: An integrative exploration of the possibilities and limits of sexual self-definition. *Journal of Psychology and Theology, 30* (2), 120-131. http://www.accessmylibrary.com

Joyce, K. (2009). *Quiverfull: Inside the Christian patriarchy movement.* Boston, MA: Beacon Press.

Kanazawa, S. (2008, April 20). *Why do boys have cooties (but brothers don't)* [Web log message]. http://www.psychologytoday.com/blog/the-scientific-fundamentalist/200804/why-boys-have-cooties-brothers-don-t

Kelly, H. C. (1954, July 2). Trends in supply of scientists and engineers in the United States. *Science, 120*(3105), 5a.

The Kinsey Institute. (n.d.). *Kinsey's heterosexual-homosexual rating scale.* http://www.kinseyinstitute.org/research/ak-hhscale.html

Kinsey Reports. (2010, February 23). In *Wikipedia.* http://en.wikipedia.org/wiki/Kinsey_Reports

Kinsey scale. (2010, March 15). In *Wikipedia.* http://en.wikipedia.org/wiki/Kinsey_scale

Kirkpatrick, R. C. (2000). The evolution of human homosexual behavior. *Current Anthropology, 41*(3), 385-413.

Klusmann, D. (n.d.). *Sperm competition and female procurement of male resources as explanations for a sex-specific time course in the sexual motivation of couples.* http://zp-m.uke.uni-hamburg.de/WebPdf/SexMot2006.pdf

Klusmann, D. (n.d.). *Sexual motivation and the duration of partnership.* http://zp-m.uke.uni-hamburg.de/Webpdf/sexmotiv.pdf

Knight, C. (2008). Early human kinship was matrilineal. In H. Callan (Ed.), *Early human kinship: From sex to social reproduction* (pp. 61-82). Hoboken, NJ: John Wiley and Sons.

Koroda, K., Miyatake, T., Nomura, Y., & Okada, K. (2008). Fighting, dispersing, and sneaking: Body-size dependent mating tactics by male Librodor japonicus beetles. *Ecological Entamology, 33,* 269-275.

LaCroix, D. (n.d.). *Lights...camera...humor! A comedy secret for a professional presentation.* http://www.fripp.com/blog/lights-camera-humor-the-rule-of-three/

Leavitt, G. C. (2007). The incest taboo? A reconsideration of Westermarck. *Anthropological Theory, 7,* 393-491. Doi: 10.1177/1463499607083427

Lee, R. B. (1993). *The Dobe Ju/'hoansi* (2nd ed) (G. & L. Spindler, Eds.). Fort Worth, TX: Harcourt College Publishers.

Legal definition of adultery. (n.d.). In *The Free Online Law Dictionary.* http://legal-dictionary.thefreedictionary.com/adultery

Lehmiller, J. J. (2018). The psychology of human sexuality. Hoboken, NJ. Wiley Blackwell.

Lewis, D. L. (2009). God's crucible: Islam and the making of Europe, 570-1215 (reprint ed.). New York, NY: W.W. Norton & Co.

LGBT Slang. (2022, February 26). In *Wikipedia.* https://en.wikipedia.org/wiki/LGBT_slang

Lloyd, E. A. (2005). *The case of the female orgasm: Bias in the science of evolution.* Cambridge, MA: Harvard University Press.

Mabe, M. (2003). The growth and number of journals. *Serials, 16*(2), 191-197.

Marriage. (1971). Merriam-Webster's Collegiate Dictionary. Merriam-Webster Incorporated.

Marriage. (1971). Simpson, J. A., Weiner, E. S. C., & Oxford University Press. The Oxford English Dictionary. Oxford: Clarendon Press.

Marriage. (2009, April 10). In *Wikipedia.* http://en.wikipedia.org/wiki/Marriage

Martel, F. (2019). *In the Closet of the Vatican.* Bloomsbury Continuum.

Martin, J. (2005). *Miss Manners' guide to excruciatingly correct behavior. Freshly updated.* New York, NY: W. W. Norton & Company.

McElvaine, R.S. (2001). *Eve's Seed: Biology, the Sexes, and the Course of History.* New York, NY. McGraw-Hill.

Meme. (2021, March 6). In *Wikipedia*. https://en.wikipedia.org/w/index.php?title=Meme&action=history

Moalem, S. (2010). *How sex works: Why we look, smell, taste, feel, and act the way we do.* New York, NY: Harper Perennial.

Monogamy. (2010, May 5). In *Wikipedia*. http://en.wikipedia.org/wiki/Monogamy

The Monogamy Puzzle. (2009, January 17). *Life Without a Net: Morality, Meaning, and Happiness Without the Crutch of Religion.* http://hambydammit.wordpress.com/2009/01/17/the-monogamy-puzzle

Morris, D. (1967). *The naked ape.* New York, NY: McGraw-Hill.

Movement Advancement Project. (2016, September). *Invisible majority: The disparities facing bisexual people and how to remedy them.* https://www.lgbtmap.org/file/invisible-majority.pdf

Multiplemoms.com. (n.d.). *Twins with different fathers.* http://en.twinshome.gov.cn/ShowNews.asp?Big_Id=3&small_Id=3&NewsId=409

Muslim World Today. (2018, July 25). *The secret history of Leviticus.* https://www.muslimworldtoday.org/the_secret_history_of_leviticus

Mustanski, B. (2010, June 8). *25-year-long study finds children with lesbian parents may be better adjusted* [Web log message]. http://www.psychologytoday.com/blog/the-sexual-continuum

National Science Foundation. (2010). *Growth rates for selected science and engineering labor force measurements.* http://www.nsf.gov/statistics/seind10/c3/c3s.htm

Nelson, R. (1994). *Babymaker: Fertility, fraud, and the fall of Doctor Cecil Jacobson.* New York, NY: Bantam Books.

Non-paternity event. (2009, March 13). In *Wikipedia*. http://en.wikipedia.org/wiki/Non-paternity_event

Office is the best bet for finding romance. (2007, May 18). http://news-for-two.cloudworth.com/local/6872.html

The origin of marriage [Web log message]. (2007, February 7). http://thearabobserver.blogspot.com/2007/02/origin-of-marriage.html

Overstreet, C. D. (2021). *Lesbian jokes of a positive nature.* Las Vegas, NV. Createspace Independent Publishing Platform.

Oxytocin. (2010, May 6). In *Wikipedia*. http://en.wikipedia.org/wiki/Oxytocin

Pacey, A. A., & Suarez, S.S. (2006). Sperm transport in the female reproductive tract. *Human Reproduction Update, 12*(1), 23-37. doi: 10.1093/humupd/dmi047

Pair-bonding: A strength and a weakness. (2008, September 24). *Reuniting: Healing with Sexual Relationships.* http://www.reuniting.info/science/pairbonding_strength_weakness

Parker, K. (2015, February 20). *Among LGBT Americans, Bisexuals Stand Out When it Comes to Identity, Acceptance.* Pew Research Center. http://pewrsr.ch/1F28

Paul, J. (n.d.). The Bisexual Identity. *Changing perspectives on sexuality: Contributions of Kinsey and anthropologists.* http://www.connexionx.org/CxLibrary/Doc/CX5017-BisexualIdentity.htm

Penn, N., & LaRose, L. (1998). *The code: Time-tested secrets for getting what you want from women – without marrying them.* New York, NY: Simon and Schuster.

Perrin, E.C. (2002, February). Technical report: Co-parent of second-parent adoption by same-sex parents. *Pediatrics, 109*(2), 341-344.

Persaud, R. (1998, December 15). *Strategy in the human pair bond.* Retrieved from http://dotpeople.com/pairbond

Peterson, M. R. (1992). *At personal risk: Boundary violations in professional-client relationships.* New York, NY: W. W. Norton.

Pew Forum on Religion and Public Life. (2008, February). *U.S. religious landscape survey. Chapter 3: Religious Affiliation and Demographic Group.* http://religions.pewforum.org/pdf/report-religious-landscape-study-chapter-3.pdf

Pew Forum on Religion and Public Life. (2010, September 28). U.S. religious knowledge survey. http://pewforum.org/U-S-Religious-Knowledge-Survey-Who-Knows-What-About-Religion.aspx

Pew Research Center. (2010). *The decline of marriage and rise of new families.* http://pew-socialtrends.org/2010/11/18/the-decline-of-marriage-and-rise-of-new-families

Pew Research Center. (2011). *91.7% – minorities account for nearly all population growth.* http://pewresearch.org/databank/dailynumber/?NumberID=1225

Pope's Westminster Hall Speech. (2010, September 17). BBC News. https;//www.bbc.com/news/uk-11352704

Population control. (2010, February 10). In *Wikipedia.* http://en.wikipedia.org/wiki/Population_control

Quinlan, R. J. (2008, September/October). Human pair-bonds: Evolutionary functions, ecological variation and adaptive development. *Evolutionary Anthropology: Issues, News, and Reviews, 17*(5), 227-238.

Riddle, K. (2010, July 4). Kids first, marriage later—if ever. *National Public Radio.* http://www.npr.org

Robinson, M. (2009, October 29). The mysteries of pair bonding [Online exclusive]. *Psychology Today.* http://www.psychologytoday.com

Robinson, M. (2009, November 10). The mysteries of pair bonding (part two) [Online exclusive]. *Psychology Today.* http://www.psychologytoday.com

Rumor has it. (2012, January 14). In *Wikipedia.* http://en.wikipedia.org/wiki/Rumor_Has_It%E2%80%A6

Ryan, C., Jetha, C. (2010) *Sex at Dawn: The Prehistoric Origins of Modern Sexuality.* New York, NY: Harper.

Same-sex marriage. (2010, November 26). In *Wikipedia.* http://en.wikipedia.org/wiki/Same-sex_marriage

Sanger, Margeret. (2022, March 7). In Wikipedia. https://en.wikipedia.org/wiki/Margaret_Sanger

Sandfort, T. G. (2005, December). Sexual orientation and gender: Stereotypes and beyond. *Archives of Sexual Behavior, 34*(6), 595-611. http://www.ncbi.nlm.nih.gov/pubmed

Sexual Script. (2010, January 23). In *Wikipedia.* http://en.wikipedia.org/wiki/Sexual_script

Shepher, J. (1971). *Self-imposed incest avoidance and exogamy in second generation Kibbutz adults* (unpublished Ph.D. thesis). Rutgers University, New Brunswick, NJ.

BIBLIOGRAPHY

Shelby, A. (2014). *The Evolution of Religion: How Religions Originate, Change, and Die.* Lexington, KY

Smil, V. (1997, July). Global Population and the Nitrogen Cycle. *Scientific American.* 76-81.

Solomon, R. C. (2006). *About love: Reinventing romance for our times.* Indianapolis, IN: Hackett Publishing Company.

Sparks, J. (1999). *Battle of the sexes: The natural history of sex.* New York, NY: TV Books, L.L.C.

Stanley, S. M. (1996). *Children of the Ice Age: How a Global Catastrophe Allowed Humans to Evolve.* Harmony Books. New York, NY.

Steiner, C. (1990). *Scripts people live: Transactional analysis of life scripts.* New York, NY: Grove Press.

Stewart, I. R. K., & Westneat, D. F. (2003, November). Extra-pair paternity in birds: Causes, correlates, and conflict. *Annual Review of Ecology, Evolution, and Systematics, 34,* 365-396.

Stone, M. (1978). *When God Was a Woman.* Boston, MA. Mariner Books.

Stookey, N. P. (1969). *The wedding song* [Musical composition].

Stuckey, J. (2005). Inanna and the "Sacred Marriage." *Matrifocus, 4* (2). http://www.matrifocus.com

Sultanoff, S. M. *What is humor?* (2010, May 19). http://www.aath.org/articles/art_sultanoff01.html

Sundaram, V. (2007, February 2). Indian feminists despair as film star marries a tree. *New America Media.* http://news.newamericamedia.org

Tattersall, I. (1998). *Becoming human: Evolution and human uniqueness.* New York, NY: Harcourt Brace & Company.

Taves, D. R. (2002, August). The intromission function of the foreskin. *Medical Hypotheses, 59*(2), 180-182. http://www.cirp.org/library

Till 2012 do us part? Mexico mulls 2-year marriage. (2011, September 29). http://today.msnbc.msn.com/id/44724855

Timeline of same-sex marriage. (March 15, 2021). In *Wikipedia.* https://en.wikipedia.org/wiki/timeline_of_same_sex_marriage.

Tonkinson, R. (1991). *The Mardu Aborigines: Living the dream in Australia's dessert* (2nd ed.) (G. & L. Spindler, Eds.). Belmont, CA: Wadsworth Group.

Types of marriages. (2010, October 18). In *Wikipedia.* http://en.wikipedia.org/wiki/Types_of_marriages

United Nations Demographic Yearbook: Focusing on Natality. (1999). *Table 13: Live Births by Legitimacy Status, and percent legitimate: 1990-1998.* http://unstats.un.org/unsd/demographic/products/dyb/dybnat.htm

U.S. Bureau of the Census. (1999). *Historical U.S. population growth by year 1900-1998.* http://www.npg.org/facts/us_historical_pops.htm

van den Berghe, P. L. (1990). *Human family systems: An evolutionary view.* Prospect Heights, IL: Waveland Press.

Varieties of monogamy. (n.d.). In *Worldlingo.* http://www.worldlingo.com/ma/enwiki/en/Varieties_of_monogamy

Vaughan, P. (2003). *The monogamy myth: A personal handbook for recovering from affairs.* (3rd ed.). New York, NY: Newmarket Press.

Vepachedu, S. (2000). *Tree marriages.* http://www.vepachedu.org

Venus Figurines. (2022, march 1). Wikipedia. https://en.wikipedia.org/wiki/Venus_-figurine

Wang, Z., & Young, L. J. (2004, October). The neurobiology of pair bonding. *Nature Neuroscience, 7*(10), 1048-1054. Doi: 10.1038/nn1327

Webster, P. (2002, August 4). Size did matter to Marie-Antoinette. *The Observer.* Guardian.co.uk/world/2002/aug/04/humanities.books

Weiner, J. (1987, March/April). When a snail leaves home. *The Sciences,* 6-10.

Westermarck, E. A. (1921). *The history of human marriage* (5th ed.). London, England: Macmillan.

Westermarck effect. (n.d.). In *Wiki.* psychology.wikia.com/wiki/Westermarck effect

Whittaker, J.C. (1994). *Flintknapping: Making and understanding stone tools.* University of Texas Press.

Wiederman, M. (2005, October). The gendered nature of sexual scripts. *The Family Journal: Counseling and Therapy for Couples and Families, 13*(4), 496-502.

Wilson, P. (2002.) Analysis: Scientists, engineers and technical workers. In *Current statistics on scientists, engineers and technical workers: 2002 edition* [Publication]. Washington, DC: Department of Professional Employees, AFL-CIO.

Wolf, S. (1998). *Guerrilla dating tactics: Strategies, tips, and secrets for finding romance.* New York, NY: Penguin Books.

Women prefer prestige over dominance in mates. (2008, December 23). *Science Daily.* http://www.sciencedaily.com/releases/2008/12/081217123825.htm

Women's choice of men goes in cycles. (1999, June 24). http://news.bbc.co.uk/2/hi/science/nature/376321.stm

World Population. (2010, March 3). In *Wikipedia.* httm://en.wikipedia.org/wiki/World_population

Wylie, K. (2007). Assessment and management of sexual problems in women. *Journal of the Royal Society of Medicine, 100,* 547-550.

INDEX

ABOUT THE AUTHOR

The author has had a long and successful career in the medical field, working in trauma centers and ERs for 40 years in various southern cities in the United States. His experiences in the ER exposed him to every conceivable aspect of human sexuality. After retiring from the ER, the author moved to Western Tennessee where he now spends his time tending to a 300-acre forest on family property and operating a small saw mill. Through his own experiences of being married and divorced twice and raising seven children, the author developed a deep curiosity about why monogamy often fails even for bright, well-educated, highly motivated people. His research led him to the surprising answers compiled in this overview of human sexual behaviors. In addition to his passion for writing, the author also enjoys timbering, fishing, hunting, and gardening.